IMMUNOLOGY AND IMMUNE SYSTEM DISORDERS

MULTIPLE SCLEROSIS

CAUSES, DIAGNOSIS AND MANAGEMENT

IMMUNOLOGY AND IMMUNE SYSTEM DISORDERS

Additional books in this series can be found on Nova's website under the Series tab.

Additional E-books in this series can be found on Nova's website under the E-books tab.

NEURODEGENERATIVE DISEASES - LABORATORY AND CLINICAL RESEARCH

Additional books in this series can be found on Nova's website under the Series tab.

Additional E-books in this series can be found on Nova's website under the E-books tab.

IMMUNOLOGY AND IMMUNE SYSTEM DISORDERS

MULTIPLE SCLEROSIS

CAUSES, DIAGNOSIS AND MANAGEMENT

ERWIN SCHOLZ
AND
CARL MÜLLER
EDITORS

Nova Science Publishers, Inc.
New York

For permission to use material from this book please contact us:
Telephone 631-231-7269; Fax 631-231-8175
Web Site: http://www.novapublishers.com

Additional color graphics may be available in the e-book version of this book.

Library of Congress Cataloging-in-Publication Data

Multiple sclerosis : causes, diagnosis, and management / editors, Erwin Scholz and Carl M|ller.
p. ; cm.
Includes bibliographical references and index.
ISBN 978-1-61324-848-5 (hardcover : alk. paper) 1. Multiple sclerosis. I. Scholz, Erwin. II. M|ller, Carl, 1974-
[DNLM: 1. Multiple Sclerosis. WL 360]
RC377.M8454 2011
616.8'34--dc23

2011018643

Published by Nova Science Publishers, Inc. † New York

Contents

Preface		**vii**
Chapter I	B Cells and Autoantibodies in Multiple Sclerosis *Klaartje Somers, Judith Fraussen, Myrthe Rouwette, Cindy Govarts, Piet Stinissen and Veerle Somers*	**1**
Chapter II	Multiple Sclerosis: The Role of Fatty Acids *Gloudina M. Hon and Tandi Matsha*	**31**
Chapter III	Multiple Sclerosis: Causes, Diagnosis and Management *Georgia Deretzi, Emmanuel Gavalas, Christos Zavos, Stergios A. Polyzos, Dimitrios Tsiptsios, Evangelia Giartza-Taxidou, Iakovos Tsiptsios and Jannis Kountouras*	**59**
Chapter IV	Epstein-Barr Virus and Multiple Sclerosis *Costanza Casiraghi and Marc S. Horwitz*	**81**
Chapter V	Actual Relation between Multiple Sclerosis and Epstein-Barr Virus *Olivia Santiago, Antonio Sorlozano, Maria José Soto, Enrique Villegas and Jose Gutierrez*	**97**
Chapter VI	MR Diffusion Tensor Imaging in Multiple Sclerosis: A Regional and Statistical Analysis of Microstructural Alterations *Dominique Sappey-Marinier, Salem Hannoun, Françoise Durand-Dubief, François Cotton and Christian Confavreux*	**113**
Chapter VII	Immunoglobulin Free Light Chains in the Diagnosis of Multiple Sclerosis *Batia Kaplan, Sizilia Golderman and Ben-Ami Sela*	**131**
Index		**143**

Preface

Multiple sclerosis is a chronic inflammatory disease of the central nervous system which leads to neuronal demyelination. As the disease progresses, oligodendrocytes and axons are destroyed, resulting in sclerotic plaques or lesion formation. Although treatment is available which can alleviate some of the symptoms, no cure is available. This book presents current research in the study of the causes, diagnosis and management of multiple sclerosis. Topics discussed include the reactivity profile of B cells and autoantibodies in MS; the role of fatty acids in neurodegenerative diseases; the possible mechanisms that the Epstein-Barr virus is exploiting to trigger MS and immunoglobulin free light chains in the diagnosis of multiple sclerosis.

Chapter I - During the last decades, investigations into MS have centered predominantly on the pathogenic role of autoreactive T cells rather than B cells. Recently, more evidence for a role of the humoral immune response in the MS pathogenesis is provided by the efficiency of novel treatment strategies; the preliminary positive results of intravenous immunoglobulin (IVIG) and B cell targeting therapy (Rituximab) in a group of MS patients have led to a renewed focus on B cells and autoantibodies in this autoimmune disease.

In this chapter, we describe the humoral immune response in MS. The B cell repertoire in healthy individuals and MS patients is discussed. Next, B cell functions in MS as well as B cell migration and survival in the central nervous system (CNS) are outlined. An overview is given of the evidence for the involvement of B cells in the pathogenesis of MS. Finally, different technologies for the study of the humoral reactivity profile in MS are described, including autoantibody profiling and B cell reactivity analysis. Phage display and B cell immortalization are described in more detail as examples of both reactivity screening approaches.

The analysis of the reactivity profile of B cells and autoantibodies in MS is relevant for the identification of novel disease markers for diagnosis, prognosis and theranostics, as well as for the elucidation of the underlying disease processes to discover highly needed novel therapeutic targets for the disease.

Chapter II- Multiple sclerosis is a chronic inflammatory disease of the central nervous system which leads to neuronal demyelination. As the disease progresses, oligodendrocytes and axons are destroyed, resulting in sclerotic plaques, or lesion formation. Although treatment is available that can alleviate some of the symptoms, no cure is available. Therefore, as more lesions are formed in the brain, nerve impulse transmission becomes progressively impaired, and brain functions are increasingly compromised, resulting in a gradual decline in health and quality of life. The underlying cause of multiple sclerosis remains unknown, but both an autoimmune and an infectious aetiology are suspected, both of which would initiate the inflammatory process. Genetic factors may also contribute to the disease aetiology. Metabolic disturbances, especially lipid metabolic abnormalities, have also been implicated in the aetiology of the disease. Although the reports are inconsistent, particularly C18:2n-6 (linoleic acid) and C20:4n-6 (arachidonic acid) have been shown to be reduced in the plasma, platelets, white and red blood cells, and CSF from patients with multiple sclerosis. These fatty acids are precursors for pro-inflammatory eicosanoid production, which are reported to be increased during the inflammatory response in neurodegenerative diseases. Eicosanoids regulate cellular functions, but their effects also depend on each precursor fatty acid and the cell type concerned. Inflammation is a defence mechanism of the body against various insults, which is usually a well-controlled process, although it may be accompanied by some damage to surrounding tissue.

Chapter III - Multiple sclerosis (MS) is an organ-specific inflammatory demyelinating disease of the central nervous system (CNS) mediated by autoreactive T lymphocytes with specificity for myelin self-antigens; it affects more than two million people worldwide and has been recognized as the leading cause of neurological disability among young adults.

MS is a multi-factorial and multigenic disorder, in which an infectious agent on a genetically permissive host can result in inflammation, demyelination and neurodegeneration. The major genetic factor in MS is the major histocompatibility complex (MHC), affecting both the immune repertoire and regulatory circuits, and the DRB*1501 allele; other susceptibility genes such as interleukin (IL)-7 and IL-2 receptors have been additionally identified. Among environmental factors such as decreased vitamin D, stress and smoking, infections are emerging as the most consistent predictors of MS risk; genes and infections by pathogens might act synergistically to trigger the disease. In this respect, the possibility that microorganisms can cause MS has recently been addressed; Epstein-Barr virus, human herpes virus-6, *Chlamydia pneumoniae*, and possibly *Helicobacter pylori* (*Hp*) may cause the neurological damage that results in MS.

Neuroinflammation might initiate from the periphery and relative data suggest that activated encephalitogenic immune effectors [T helper cell (Th)1, Th17, CD8 cells, B cells, and macrophages], through the disrupted blood-brain barrier, powerfully influence the processes in the brain. Active inflammation, marked by augmented numbers of activated and primed microglia, increased steady-state levels of inflammatory cytokines and decreases in anti-inflammatory molecules, may determine the initial phase of the disease. In the CNS, an immunological cascade, consisting of epitope spreading, triggers the activation of the innate immune system (microglia, dendritic cells, astrocytes, B cells), which leads to chronic inflammation. Demyelination is observed in both white and gray matter of the CNS. Four different pathological patterns (Lassmann's patterns) have been identified in the lesions in the brain tissue (pattern I: T-cell-mediated; pattern II: T-cell plus antibody-mediated autoimmune response; patterns III and IV: highly suggestive of a primary oligodendrocyte dystrophy).

Several clinical forms of MS have been described such as relapsing-remitting MS (RRMS), secondary progressive, primary progressive and progressive-relapsing. This classification is important both for prognosis and therapeutic decisions. RRMS is characterized by unpredictable relapses followed by periods of remission. Approximately

10% of patients begin with a primary progressive form of the disease being the most disabling.

MS symptoms develop as the cumulative result of multiple lesions in the brain and spinal cord. Neurological symptoms include visual problems, changes in sensation, muscle weakness, ataxia, fatigue, bladder and bowel difficulties, cognitive impairment and emotional symptoms.

Diagnosis is based on the McDonald criteria focusing on clinical, laboratory and radiologic data of the dissemination MS lesions in time and space. The most commonly used diagnostic tools are magnetic resonance imaging, analysis of the cerebrospinal fluid for oligoclonal bands of immunoglobulin G and evoked potential.

Although the cure of MS is unknown, a multidisciplinary approach has proven to be helpful. Management aims to restore the function after a relapse (using intravenous administration of high doses of corticosteroids) and to prevent new relapses and disability (using disease-modifying treatments or immunosuppressors). MS medications and rehabilitation programs (physiotherapy, neurocognitive and psychological rehabilitation) improve the quality of life of MS patients. Expectedly, *Hp* eradication might alter the initiation and/or progression of MS.

Chapter IV- Multiple sclerosis (MS) is an immune-mediated disease of the central nervous system that leads to myelin loss and progressive disability. The causes of MS are still unknown but the disease process is likely triggered by an environmental factor(s) in genetically susceptible individuals. Several different viruses have been identified as possible MS triggers but increasing evidence strongly associates Epstein-Barr virus (EBV) to MS. Epidemiological findings show that EBV infection, especially if accompanied by mononucleosis, greatly increases MS risk. Other relevant findings include the correlation between disease onset and the titer of anti-EBV antibodies in the serum. Dysregulated EBV specific T cells responses have been detected in MS, suggesting that MS patients might have a decreased ability to control EBV replication and there is also evidence of cross-reactivity between EBV antigens and myelin. The main site of EBV latency is the B cell compartment and B cell depletion therapies have been recently shown to strongly reduce disease activity in relapsing-remitting MS. Intriguingly EBV positive B cell follicles have been found in the brain of MS patients. Further, EBV has been shown to infect cell types other than B cells and these could play a role in MS pathogenesis. Despite all these findings, it is still unclear how EBV triggers MS. In this review we will summarize past literature and discuss possible mechanisms that EBV is exploiting to trigger MS.

Chapter V - Multiple sclerosis is a demyelinating disease that affects the central nervous system and one of the most common causes of neurologic disability in young adults. Although its pathogenesis is not clear, it seems to have an immune basis in genetically-sensitive persons. Some factors, most of them still unknown, may trigger the activation of the immune system to produce inflammatory damages that may include demyelination, axonal damages and oligodendrocyte loss, followed by structural repair, post-inflammatory gliosis and neurodegeneration.

Over the past 50 years, a great number of work groups have researched the possible participation of infectious agents in multiple sclerosis, and a significant number of microorganisms have been proposed as possible candidates in the pathogenesis of this inflammatory and demyelinating process. Amongst the numerous candidate microorganisms, many publications have linked viruses from the *Herpesviridae* family, especially, the Epstein-Barr virus, to the disease.

Several hypotheses have been proposed in an attempt to explain the role of this virus. That is the case of the molecular mimetic hypothesis, infection of autoimmune B-cells, superantigen and αB-crystallin protein, or the hygiene hypothesis. Nonetheless, the diversity of results obtained shows the need for an analytic summary of the findings of all the scientific literature available in order to integrate them and establish whether there is any real evidence of an association between infection and disease, defining a possible theoretical framework on the scientific knowledge available on the issue that may subsequently be useful in clinical practice and health care.

Chapter VI - Magnetic Resonance Imaging (MRI) became the first radiological examination that is essential to the diagnosis of Multiple Sclerosis (MS), and most informative for the understanding of the illness and the patient care. If conventional MRI shows the lesion load reflecting mainly the inflammatory aspect of the disease, the lack of clinico-radiological correlation has led to the research of new markers for monitoring and predicting the progression of the disease to better adapt the medical treatment to each patient. Therefore, quantitative MR methods have been developed to better access these alterations that were undetectable by conventional MRI such as diffusion tensor imaging (DTI). DTI is a very promising technique for fiber tracking the cerebral white matter (WM) as well as to provide accurate quantification of biophysic markers reflecting microstructure alterations of axonal/neuronal integrity and connectivity. This information can be obtained through the measurement of several parameters such as the fractional anisotropy (FA), the mean diffusivity (MD) and the axial and radial diffusivities (λa and λr) by selecting regions of interest (ROI) in lesions, normal appearing WM or structures such as the corpus callosum. More recently, the ability to analyze DTI data in a voxelwise approach using statistic techniques such "Tract-Based Spatial Statistics" (TBSS) allowed us to localize alterations in an observer-independent manner in the whole WM of patients with different clinical forms.

Therefore, to investigate the role of DTI for better characterizing the pathological processes in different clinical forms of MS, we performed a study on 69 patients with Relapsing Remitting (RR), primary (PP) and secondary progressive (SP) and 29 control subjects. The quantification of DTI metrics demonstrated significant increases of MD, λa, and λr, and a decrease of FA in MS patients of any clinical form compared to control subjects. Moreover, these alterations were significantly greater in progressive forms such SP and PP compared to RR. Compared to FA and λa, the radial diffusivity showed the best sensitivity to detect alterations. This result may suggest a better specificity of this marker to the demyelinating and inflammatory processes. As shown by both ROI and TBSS approaches, the corpus callosum appeared the most and earliest damaged structure in RR patients, probably due to inflammatory attacks as confirmed by the good correlation obtained between DTI values and the lesion load. Therefore, DTI metrics constitute an early and sensitive marker to follow-up the white matter alterations and better understand the disease progression.

Chapter VII - The diagnosis of multiple sclerosis (MS) is based on clinical criteria, magnetic resonance imaging (MRI) data and laboratory findings. The latter include information obtainable from analysis of cerebrospinal fluid (CSF) where demonstration of oligoclonal immunoglobulin G (IgG) bands (OCB) indicates an intrathecal production of IgGs and supports diagnosis of MS. One of the major disadvantages of this commonly used test is that OCBs might be detected in other inflammatory and infectious diseases of the central nervous system. Thus, search for novel technologies and new MS-specific markers is of diagnostic value.

This review highlights the potential importance of Ig free light chains (FLCs) as novel diagnostic markers for MS. Different methods applied to analyze FLCs in the CSF of MS patients are described. These include immunochemical methods based on electrophoretic techniques, as well as radioimmunoassay and nephelometric immunoassay. Application of these methods brought valuable information with regard to the characteristic features of FLCs in MS: κ and λ level, their oligoclonality and monomer-dimer patterns. In this review, the advantages and disadvantages of the reported methods are discussed with respect to their specificity, sensitivity, complexity and availability. While none of the reported methods is perfect, many of them may complement each other by providing a more comprehensive characterization of FLCs in MS. Considering the heterogeneous nature of MS, such information may assist in further studies aimed to establish new laboratory markers for different forms and stages of this disease.

In: Multiple Sclerosis
Editor: E. Scholz and C. Müller, pp. 1-30
ISBN 978-1-61324-848-5

Chapter I

B Cells and Autoantibodies in Multiple Sclerosis

Klaartje Somers[1,*,†], Judith Fraussen[1,†], Myrthe Rouwette[1], Cindy Govarts[1], Piet Stinissen[1] and Veerle Somers[1]
Hasselt University, Biomedical Research Institute, Agoralaan, building C, 3590 Diepenbeek, Belgium

Abstract

During the last decades, investigations into MS have centered predominantly on the pathogenic role of autoreactive T cells rather than B cells. Recently, more evidence for a role of the humoral immune response in the MS pathogenesis is provided by the efficiency of novel treatment strategies; the preliminary positive results of intravenous immunoglobulin (IVIG) and B cell targeting therapy (Rituximab) in a group of MS patients have led to a renewed focus on B cells and autoantibodies in this autoimmune disease.

In this chapter, we describe the humoral immune response in MS. The B cell repertoire in healthy individuals and MS patients is discussed. Next, B cell functions in MS as well as B cell migration and survival in the central nervous system (CNS) are outlined. An overview is given of the evidence for the involvement of B cells in the pathogenesis of MS. Finally, different technologies for the study of the humoral reactivity profile in MS are described, including autoantibody profiling and B cell reactivity analysis. Phage display and B cell immortalization are described in more detail as examples of both reactivity screening approaches.

The analysis of the reactivity profile of B cells and autoantibodies in MS is relevant for the identification of novel disease markers for diagnosis, prognosis and theranostics, as well as for the elucidation of the underlying disease processes to discover highly needed novel therapeutic targets for the disease.

* Corresponding author: Veerle Somers, Hasselt University, Biomedical Research Institute, Agoralaan, building C, 3590 Diepenbeek, Belgium, tel. +3211269202, email: veerle.somers@uhasselt.be.

† Both authors contributed equally.

Multiple sclerosis (MS) has been regarded as a T cell mediated disorder for a long time. This focus on T cells was partly attributed to the long-standing observation that an important lymphocytic subset in MS lesions was composed of T cells [1]. In addition, the clear pathogenic effect of myelin-reactive T cells in the animal model of MS, experimental autoimmune encephalomyelitis (EAE), contributed to the belief that autoreactive T cells were at the center of the MS pathogenic processes [2]. Recent studies into B cell and antibody-depleting therapeutic strategies in MS have renewed interest into the involvement of B cells in the underlying disease pathogenesis [3-6]. During the last decades, more and more evidence has been collected for an important role of the humoral immune response in MS pathogenesis.

In this chapter, the B cell repertoire in healthy individuals and MS patients will first be discussed. Next, B cell functions in MS, B cell migration and survival in the central nervous system (CNS) are outlined. An overview is given of the evidence for the involvement of B cells in the pathogenesis of MS. Finally, different technologies for the study of the humoral reactivity profile in MS are described.

1. The B Cell Repertoire in Healthy Individuals and MS Patients

In order to examine the role of B cells in the pathogenesis of MS, it is important to understand the B cell maturation process. The distribution of the different B cell subpopulations that make up the B cell repertoire in healthy individuals and MS patients has already been thoroughly analyzed.

1.1. B Cell Maturation

Mature naïve B cells, which are characterized by expression of the general B cell marker CD19 and the absence of CD27 and CD38 on their surface [7], are released in the peripheral blood after development in the bone marrow and secondary lymphoid organs [8;9]. Recognition of an antigen in lymphoid tissue triggers B cell activation, which is accompanied by an upregulation of CD80 and CD86 surface expression. After activation, B cells proliferate into plasma blasts that produce low-affinity antibody for a few days [10] or further differentiate into different effector B cell subtypes in germinal centers (GC) via the centrocyte and centroblast stages [11]. This differentiation is accompanied by an upregulation of CD38 surface expression [12-14]. In this case, memory B cells, plasma blasts or plasma cells are developed after extensive mutation and maturation [15;16]. Memory B cells, expressing both CD19 and the memory surface marker CD27 [7], are able to reactivate and differentiate into plasma cells very fast upon a new challenge with their antigen. Plasma cells have lost proliferating capacity and are mostly long-lived antibody-producing cells that no longer display CD19 but do express CD38, CD138 and CD27. Plasma blasts, on the other hand, are short-lived antibody-secreting cells expressing CD19, CD27, CD38 but also the plasma cell marker CD138.

1.2. B Cell Repertoire in Healthy Individuals and MS Patients

In healthy individuals, most B cells that populate the peripheral blood belong to the naïve B cell population, although some circulating memory B cells can be denoted. The antibody-secreting effector cells move into the target tissues to eliminate their target cells and consequently cannot be found in the blood. B cells are rarely found in the cerebrospinal fluid (CSF) of healthy persons and patients with a non-inflammatory neurological disease (NIND) [16].

The peripheral blood of MS patients displays a similar B cell subtype distribution as that of healthy individuals, mostly harbouring B cells with a $CD19^+CD27^-$ naïve phenotype [17;18]. The CSF of MS patients and patients with other inflammatory neurological disorders (OIND) contains on average 4-5% of $CD19^+$ B cells, opposite to the situation in healthy persons. Variability in CSF B cell numbers was seen between patients [16;17;19-21], but the majority were mature $CD19^+CD27^+CD38^-CD138^-$ memory B cells [17;18;22]. $CD19^+CD38^{high}CD77^+$ $Ki67^+Bcl\text{-}2^-$ centroblasts, that normally only occur in GC in lymphatic tissues [23], were demonstrated in the CSF [16;18], either as the result of circulating memory B cell recruitment to the CNS or intrathecal differentiation of naïve B cells. Both processes can be promoted by ectopic GC that were identified in the meninges of MS patients and suggest that antibody-secreting cells can be generated within the CNS [24].

Table 1. Overview B cell subsets in healthy individuals and MS: expression of surface markers and distribution in periphery and CSF

	naïve B cell	memory B cell	plasma blast	centroblast	plasma cell	references
surface markers	$CD19^+$ $CD27^-$ $CD38^-$	$CD19^+$ $CD27^+$ $CD138^-$ $CD38^-$	$CD19^+$ $CD27^{high}$ $CD138^+$ $CD38^+$	$CD19^+$ $CD77^+$ $Ki67^+$ $Bcl\text{-}2^-$ $CD38^{high}$	$CD19^-$ $CD27^{high}$ $CD138^+$ $CD38^+$	[16-19;25;27]
healthy persons						
periphery	+	(+)	-	-	-	[18;26]
CSF	-	-	-	-	-	[17;20;28]
multiple sclerosis						
periphery	+	(+)	-	-	-	[17;18;20;28]
CSF	-	+	+	+	+/(+)	[16-21;25;28]

+ present; - not present; (+) present in low amounts.

Plasma blasts ($CD19^+CD38^+CD138^+$) have also been described as an important CSF B cell population. Numbers of plasma blasts were significantly increased in CSF of patients with MS and clinically isolated syndrome (CIS), a first (sub)acute neurological event with demyelination, when compared with OIND patients [20]. Furthermore, the number of mature memory B cells and plasma blasts in the CSF of MS patients was correlated with intrathecal immunoglobulin G (IgG) and immunoglobulin M (IgM) production, higher disease activity and lesions on magnetic resonance imaging (MRI), total CSF leukocyte numbers and intrathecal production of MMP-9 (matrix metalloproteinase 9), and the homing chemokine CXCL-13 (chemokine (C-X-C motif) ligand 13) [17;20]. These findings all indicate that CSF B cells play a role in acute inflammation. Being the most prevalent antibody-secreting cells in the CSF, plasma blasts are held responsible for intrathecal IgG production and are consequently mentioned as main effector B cell population in acute inflammation in MS [17]. Normally, plasma blasts are short-lived antibody-secreting cells that rapidly differentiate into fully mature $CD19^{-}CD138^{+}$ plasma cells. In MS, however, plasma blast numbers remained virtually constant over time [17], which might demonstrate an antigen-driven chronic B cell stimulation in the CNS.

Disagreement exists concerning the contribution of $CD19^{-}CD38^{+}CD138^{+}$ plasma cells to the B cell repertoire in the CSF compartment. While some studies pointed out very low numbers of plasma cells [17;20;25], another study demonstrated a high number of plasma cells in the CSF of MS patients [18]. Nevertheless, the distribution of plasma blasts and plasma cells in the CSF remains vague, although $CD19^{+}CD138^{+}$ and $CD19^{-}CD138^{+}$ cells have recently been shown to be derived from the same progenitor pool and thus represent convergent responses [25]. The absence of plasma cells in the CSF of MS patients in some studies could be explained by the fact that plasma cells migrate to the brain meninges and parenchyma so they are hard to detect in CSF. Moreover, surface marker expression profiles have not been entirely clarified for plasma cells and plasma blasts. Previously, it has even been shown that CD138 was not expressed on the surface of plasma blasts and consequently was the only surface marker allowing to differentiate between plasma cells and plasma blasts [26]. Thus the phenotypic differences between these two cell types still have to be determined in detail. Table 1 gives an overview of the different B cell subsets, their surface marker expression profiles and distribution among peripheral blood and CSF.

2. Functions of B cells in MS Pathogenesis

2.1. Antibody Dependent Functions

B cells in MS have traditionally been associated with the production of autoantibodies. Plasma cells and plasma blasts in the CNS generate antibodies that recognize self antigens. These pathogenic antibodies can clear target cells via antibody-dependent cell-mediated cytotoxicity (ADCC) or complement activation (Fig. 1-1) [29-31]. In ADCC, autoantibodies bind Fc receptors on macrophages, neutrophils and natural killer (NK) cells that consequently attack myelin by phagocytosis. This further leads to activation of phagocyte oxidase and secretion of hydrolytic enzymes that induce tissue damage and inflammation [31]. Alternatively, autoantibodies bind directly to their target antigen and activate the complement cascade through complement fixation. The Fc region of the antibody binds to complement component C1q, resulting in activation of the complement cascade. This ultimately leads to the generation of a membrane attack complex (MAC) that is inserted into the cell membrane of the target cell to cause lysis and cell death [31;32].

2.2. Antibody Independent Functions

B cells exert antibody independent functions in MS pathogenesis as well. B cells secrete proinflammatory cytokines, such as interleukin-6 (IL-6) and tumor necrosis factor (TNF), that enhance tissue damage in the CNS by activation of macrophages and T cells (Fig. 1-2) [33]. These cytokines can modulate the migration of dendritic cells and provide feedback stimulatory signals for further B cell activation [30]. The immunosuppressive cytokine interleukin-10 (IL-10) is produced as well, and is more important in dampening of the immune response [16;34]. Although their antigen presenting capacity is low when capturing antigen in a nonspecific manner, B cells are potent antigen-presenting cells (APC) for the activation of T cells of the same specificity [35;36]. In this way, B cells participate in the generation and maintenance of T cell clonal expansion and cytokine production (Fig. 1-3). In addition, B cells provide co-stimulation in the T cell activation process (Fig. 1-4) [29;34]. Increase in the number of circulating B cells that express the costimulatory receptors CD80 (cluster of differentiation 80) and CD86 (B7-1) again contributes to T cell clonal expansion and cytokine production [37;38]. Furthermore, B cells are involved in the formation and maintenance of ectopic lymphoid follicles (Fig. 1-5), large B cell aggregates in the meninges of MS patients. The formation of such follicular structures is driven by dendritic cells and B cells through the actions of cytokines and chemokines including CXCL-12, CXCL-13 and lymphotoxin [18]. Finally, B cells in MS produce neurotrophic factors such as nerve growth factor [39], brain-derived neurotrophic factor [40] and neurturin [41]. These might help in restoring CNS integrity.

3. B Cell Migration and Survival in the CNS

Migration of B cells to the brain is directed by CXCL-13, CXCL-10 and CXCL-12 that are secreted by endothelial cells and are upregulated in the brain of MS patients [16;42;43]. In addition, migration is facilitated by very late antigen-4 (VLA-4) and lymphocyte function-associated antigen-1 (LFA-1) [42]. These adhesion molecules bind to vascular cell adhesion molecule-1 (VCAM-1) and intercellular adhesion molecule-1 (ICAM-1) on endothelial cells to direct B cells from the circulation into the CNS.

BAFF (B cell activating factor of the TNF family, tumor necrosis factor ligand superfamily member 13B) and A proliferation inducing ligand (APRIL) are two important regulators of B cell survival and activation in the CNS, but also of differentiation, GC formation and Ig production [44;45]. Both members of the TNF family are produced by monocytes, macrophages and dendritic cells [30]. Their receptors on the B cell surface are BAFF-receptor (BAFF-R), B cell maturation antigen (BCMA) and transmembrane activator and calcium modulator and cytophilin ligand interactor (TACI) [45]. BAFF may synergize with CXCL-12, CXCL-13 and CCL-19 (chemokine (C-C motif) ligand 19) to attract and maintain B cells in the inflamed CNS of MS patients [46]. Levels of BAFF, BAFF-R and APRIL messenger RNA (mRNA) are increased in patients with MS, where they are produced by astrocytes [47-49]. The group of Serafini recently reported strong BAFF immunoreactivity in infiltrating Epstein-Barr virus (EBV)-infected B cells that were organized in ectopic B cell follicles in the meninges of MS brains [50]. BAFF and APRIL have furthermore been described to be relevant targets for therapy of various autoimmune disorders and could be used in that context since intravenous Ig contains anti-BAFF and anti-APRIL antibodies [15;51].

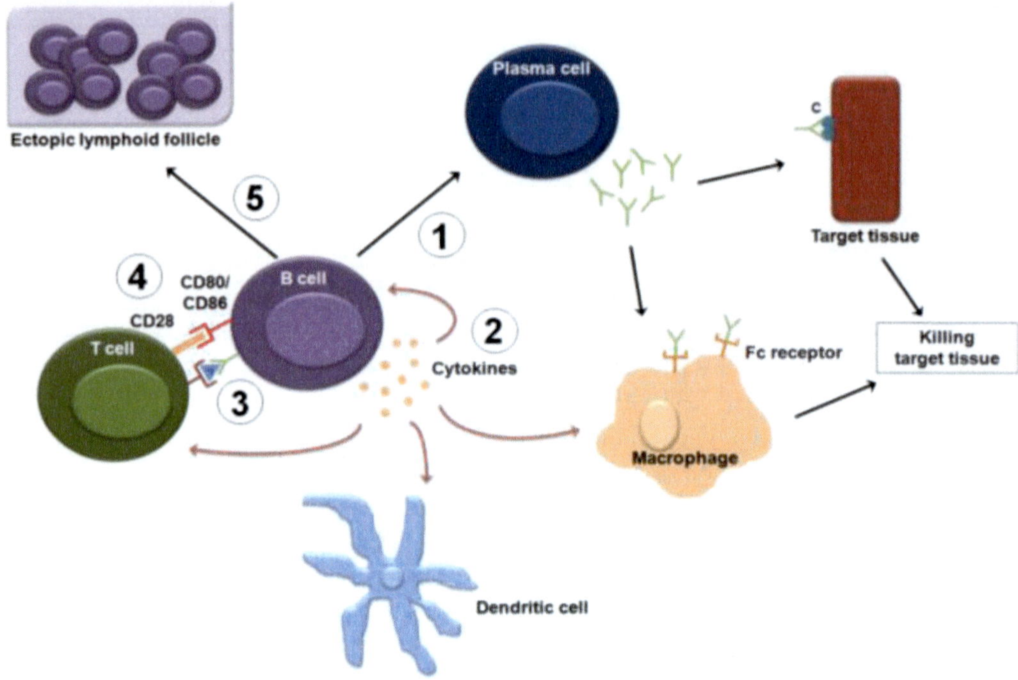

Figure 1. Functions of B cells in MS. (1) Production of (auto)antibodies that cause killing of their target tissue by antibody-dependent cell-mediated cytotoxicity (ADCC) or by complement activation. (2) Secretion of proinflammatory cytokines, such as TNF and IL-6, activate macrophages, T cells and dendritic cells to enhance tissue damage. They also provide positive feedback signals for further B cell activation. Production of IL-10 by B cells causes suppression of the immune response. (3) B cells function as antigen-presenting cells, which results in T cell clonal expansion and cytokine production. (4) B cells provide costimulatory signals during T cell activation. B7 molecules (CD80 or CD86) on B cells bind to CD28 on the T cell surface to provide this costimulation. (5) Formation and maintenance of ectopic GC in the meninges. Abbreviation: c, complement.

4. Evidence for a Role of B Cells and Autoantibodies in MS Pathogenesis

The first evidence for the presence of a distorted humoral immune response was already detected a long time ago: oligoclonal immunoglobulin (Ig) bands (OCB) were described by Elvin Kabat in 1948 and by EC Laterre in 1964 as being composed of increased Ig generated by antibody-secreting cells in the CNS, thus indicating an intrathecal Ig production in MS [52;53]. At least 2 OCB are present in the CSF that are not present in the corresponding serum sample [54;55]. Two or more OCB exclusive to the CSF are detected in more than 95% of MS patients [56;57] and presence of OCB even constitutes one of the diagnostic criteria for MS [58]. Analysis of the Ig genes of B cells in the CSF and MS lesions confirmed the presence of an intrathecal, antigen-driven, affinity-matured B cell response [59;60].

In addition, B cells, plasma cells, plasma blasts and myelin-binding antibodies have been reported in MS lesions and MS CSF [61-64]. Pattern II demyelinating lesions, characterized by Ig deposits and involvement of the complement system, are furthermore the most frequent (approximately 58%) lesion type in MS patients [65]. B cell cytokines, such as BAFF, were also detected in MS lesions [47]. Ectopic lymphoid follicles containing proliferating B cells and plasma cells have recently been demonstrated in the meninges of a subset of MS patients [66;67]. These are large B cell aggregates consisting primarily of memory B cells that are localized in the sub-arachnoid space, mainly inside the cerebral sulci and display several features of germinal centers including the presence of dendritic cells expressing CXCL13, B cell proliferation, expression of activation-induced cytidine deaminase and plasma cell differentiation [68]. Ectopic lymphoid follicles have also been denoted in EAE [69]. Moreover, the presence of a distorted humoral immune response in MS was shown to be associated with a worse disease outcome [70], while findings in EAE supported an important role of the humoral autoimmune response in disease pathology. Passive antibody transfer experiments with antibodies directed against myelin oligodendrocyte glycoprotein (MOG) at the onset of acute EAE in rat resulted in extensive plaque-like demyelination and exacerbation of the clinical signs [71]. For the first time, this study provided clear evidence for the demyelinating capacity of antibodies. Subsequent studies showed that antibodies directed against other prevalent myelin components such as myelin basic protein (MBP) and galactocerebroside (Galc) or neuronal components such as neurofascin also could have an effect on the EAE disease course [72;73]. Besides the role of CNS-reactive antibodies in EAE, B cells have been shown to be required for disease induction in several EAE models (reviewed in [74]). Recently, more conclusive evidence for a role of the humoral immune response in MS pathogenesis has been provided by the efficiency of novel treatment strategies; the preliminary positive results of intravenous immunoglobulin (IVIG) and B cell depleting therapy (Rituximab) in a group of MS patients have led to a renewed focus on B cells and autoantibodies in this autoimmune disease [75-77].

On the other hand, besides evidence for a pathogenic role of the humoral immune response in MS, there are also indications that B cell cytokines, neurotrophic factors and antibodies might downregulate immune responses and promote repair and remyelination. These findings point towards a beneficial effect of the humoral immune response in the MS disease process [78-80].

The above findings support an important role of B cells in MS. Whether B cells are implicated in disease initiation or whether their involvement is secondary to the causative immune response is still not clear (reviewed in [81]). Further analysis of the antigen reactivity of B cells in MS is warranted to obtain more information regarding the underlying disease processes.

5. Analysis of the Humoral Reactivity Profile in MS

Numerous approaches are currently used to investigate reactivity of the humoral immune response with different success rates, and despite a lot of effort the targets of the autoreactive B cells and antibodies are not yet known. Since MS is characterized by a heterogeneous disease course and genetic background, novel markers for the diagnosis of patients and a multiplex treatment strategy are needed for better control of the disease. Studying the humoral immune response thus remains a hot topic in MS research where identification of the target antigens is one of the main goals. Different approaches for reactivity analysis of the humoral immune response in MS are discussed below. Phage display and B cell immortalization technology are described in more detail.

CSF can be a useful surrogate for the brain microenvironment and is therefore suitable to study antibody responses in MS. Moreover, oligoclonal Ig have mainly been described in the CSF of MS patients. However, CSF may also comprise antibodies originating from the peripheral blood that are not specific to the disease. Disease-relevant autoreactive antibodies may even bind to their targets or to Fc receptors in the CNS tissue, rendering them undetectable in CSF. Serum can be used as an alternative to study B cell reactivity in MS. Intrathecally produced antibodies are able to diffuse from the CSF into the circulation, leaving them detectable in the serum. In addition, several studies have described the increased presence of specific antibody reactivity in serum of MS patients when compared to neurological controls, demonstrating that serum autoantibody profiles can be used to distinguish MS patients from control subjects [82-84].

Most studies investigating the specificity of the humoral immune response have focused on autoantibodies directly by analyzing reactivity of the antibodies in serum or CSF of MS patients versus healthy controls or other neurological control patients. A substantial amount of the already identified candidate autoantigens have been denoted in this way. An alternative approach that does not suffer from binding of antibodies to their target antigens or from dilution and breakdown of antibodies, would be to investigate the reactivity of the expanded (autoreactive) B cells in MS. The main findings of both reactivity profiling approaches in MS are described below.

5.1. Autoantibody Profiling in MS

In the past, different experimental approaches have been used for analysis of the autoantibody specificities in the serum and CSF of MS patients. Table 2 contains a summary of all previously reported antigenic targets of autoantibodies in MS (reviewed in [85;86]). As it is thought that in MS, the myelin in the CNS is the primary target of the aberrant autoimmune response, different myelin components were firstly proposed as candidate autoantigens (Table 2). There are numerous reports about antibodies directed against MBP [87], MOG [88], proteolipid protein (PLP) [89] and myelin-associated glycoprotein (MAG) [90] in MS patients but up till now, none of these myelin-associated candidate antigens definitely discriminates between the humoral immune response in MS patients and healthy controls [91-94]. The true relevance of anti-myelin antibodies in the MS disease process and in the development of MS disease markers remains inconclusive. Moreover, other CNS-specific components such as neuronal, axonal and glial compounds have been analyzed as autoantibody targets in MS (Table 2) [95;96]. There are however also reports about the presence of antibodies against more ubiquitous *self*-antigens such as heat-shock proteins (hsp) [97] and DNA (deoxyribonucleic acid) [98] (Table 2).

Up till now, the reported sensitivities and specificities of the identified individual autoantibodies for MS are at best only moderate. Not one of the autoantibodies is specifically present only in MS patients. Moreover, all autoantibodies are present in a subpopulation of

MS patients. This can be explained by the enormous heterogeneity which is characteristic for MS and is reflected in the diversity of MS disease courses, treatment efficiencies and prevailing pathogenic processes.

5.1.1. Multiplexing Approaches for Autoantibody Profiling in MS

In recent years, the need for multiplex autoantibody profiling approaches has become evident within the research domain of autoimmunity [99;100], since autoimmune diseases are characterized by broad autoantibody profiles with considerable overlap between the different diseases [101;102]. This overlap in reactivity profile and the heterogeneous nature of MS, represented in the diversity of disease courses, treatment efficiencies and prevailing pathogenic processes, underscore the importance of a multiplexing approach to fully elucidate the MS autoantibody profile. The identification of a MS-specific autoantibody fingerprint can be of great use from a diagnostic point of view, but can also provide valuable information regarding disease-specific humoral immune responses and thus the underlying autoimmune aetiology and pathogenesis.

Different multiplexing approaches such as the use of antigen microarrays, high-throughput blotting procedures and lambda phage expression library screening, have already been used for the identification of a disease-specific autoantibody fingerprint in MS serum and MS CSF.

By application of lipid-antigen microarrays for autoantibody profiling in MS CSF, Kanter *et al.* demonstrated increased lipid-specific antibody reactivity against different myelin lipids including sulfatide, sphingomyelin, oxidized lipids and microbial lipids in individuals with MS [103]. Based on a similar microarray technology, Quintana *et al.* recently reported the identification of unique serum autoantibody patterns that distinguished relapsing-remitting MS (RRMS), secondary progressive MS (SPMS) and primary progressive MS (PPMS) patients from each other and from healthy controls (HC) and patients with other neurological and autoimmune diseases [104]. Moreover, patients with different immunopathologic patterns of MS (based on brain biopsy analysis) could be discerned based on unique autoantibody profiles [105]. However, despite the interesting results obtained, the main drawback of antigen array screening is the fact that it is a so-called biased autoantibody profiling approach; only a small number of known and characterized antigens are spotted as candidate antigenic targets, which is not fully representative for the heterogeneity present within the *in vivo* target tissue in MS, namely the inflamed CNS. Moreover, by applying this approach, the identification of novel antigenic targets is not possible.

An alternative, less biased protein array system for autoantibody profiling in MS was applied by the research group of Hemmer [106]. Protein arrays were prepared by the spotting of 37,000 different expression clones, obtained from a human fetal brain complementary DNA (cDNA) library. Probing of these arrays with individual CSF samples from MS and control patients resulted in the identification of two EBV proteins (Table 2) against which significantly higher serum and CSF immunoreactivities were identified in MS patients [107].

Several research groups have applied more unbiased proteomics approaches to elucidate MS autoantibody profiles. Lefranc *et al.* identified distinct serum IgG antibody repertoires against human brain homogenates between MS patients and control subjects by application of 1-D (1 dimensional) and 2-D (2 dimensional) immunoblotting techniques [108]. Furthermore, specific IgG reactivity profiles that could discriminate between the three forms of MS (RR, SP and PP) were detected [109].

Table 2. MS antibody reactivities

Myelin antigens (proteins, glycoproteins and lipids)	
Myelin oligodendrocyte glycoprotein	[115]
Myelin basic protein	[116;117]
Myelin associated glycoprotein	[118]
Proteolipid protein	[119]
CSF114(Glc)	[120]
Glc(alpha1,4)Glc(alpha)	[121]
Myelin lipids (phosphatidylcholine, sulfatide, sphingomyelin)	[122;123]
Galactocerebroside	[124]
Cerebellar soluble lectin	[125]
Axonal and neuronal antigens	
Neurofilaments (light and medium chain)	[126]
Gangliosides (GD1a, GM3, sulfatide)	[127]
Axolemma-Enriched Fraction	[128]
Tubulin	[129]
Nogo-A	[130]
Nogo receptor	[131]
Surface antigen on neuronal cell line	[132]
Neurofascin 186	[133]
Contactin-2	[134]
Oligodendrocyte antigens	
Surface antigen on oligodendrocyte-precursor derived cell line	[135]
Oligodendrocyte progenitor cell-specific surface glycoprotein	[136]
Oligodendrocyte-specific protein	[137]
Transaldolase	[138]
2',3'-cyclic nucleotide 3' phosphodiesterase	[139]
Stress proteins	
Alpha-B-crystallin	[140]
Hsp60	[141]
Hsp70	[142]
Hsp90β	[143]
Ubiquitous and other antigens	
Proteasome	[144]
DNA	[145]
Heterogeneous nuclear ribonucleoprotein B1	[146]
Retinal arrestin	[147]
Triosephosphate isomerase	[148]
Glyceraldehyde 3-phosphate dehydrogenase	[149]
Alu-peptide	[150]
Epstein-Barr nuclear antigen 1	[151]
BRRF2 (EBV protein)	[152]

Based on [153;154].

An analogous 1-D immunoblotting procedure of human brain lysates with purified MS CSF IgG by Kolln *et al.* led to the identification of triosephosphate isomerase (TPI) and glyceraldehyde 3-phosphate dehydrogenase (GAPDH) as MS CSF antibody targets (Table 2) [110]. A similar proteomics approach was applied by the research groups of Linington and Meinl. In this study, serum and Ig preparations from MS and control patients were used in 1-D and 2-D blotting experiments of glycoproteins isolated from human myelin by lentil-lectin affinity chromatography [111;112]. These experiments led to the identification of 2 novel and promising antibody-targets in MS patients, namely neurofascin and contactin-2 (Table 2) [113;114].

The application of immunoblotting of brain preparations for autoantibody profiling allows the identification of novel antigenic targets. In addition, the *in vivo* antigenic composition of the diseased tissue is conserved to a higher extent in this immunoblotting procedure. Drawbacks of the technology are the relatively low sensitivity (especially for less abundant proteins) and the inherent biases in antigen representation due to use of denaturing polyacrylamide gel electrophoresis.

Archelos *et al.* compared pooled CSF from MS patients with that from patients with other neurological diseases by applying a high-throughput filter screening procedure on a lambda phage cDNA expression library constructed from an oligodendrocyte-precursor cell [155]. A sequence motif of 7 amino acids that was homologous to a translated consensus Alu repeat epitope was detected and further analysis showed that 44% of MS sera and CSF reacted with these Alu-peptides (Table 1.1) [156].

Similar screenings of lambda phage expression libraries constructed from chronic MS plaques with MS CSF and MS serum by Owens *et al.* did not result in the identification of MS-specific target antigens [157].

5.1.2. Autoantibody Profiling with Phage Display Technology

More than 20 years ago, phage display technology using filamentous phage was developed by Smith [158]. The technique is based on the ability of phage virions, virus particles that infect and amplify in bacteria, to incorporate foreign DNA into their genome, coupled to a gene encoding a phage coat protein [159;160]. After infection, phage protein components are produced by the protein translation machinery of the infected bacterial host cell and the incorporated DNA is translated into the corresponding DNA product, covalently coupled to the phage coat protein. Upon phage virion assembly, the recombinant coat protein will be incorporated into the virion protein coat [160]. The (poly)peptide product, encoded by the DNA insert, is displayed at the surface of the phage particle and is thus available for experimental strategies. The strength of the phage display technology lies within the physical link

between DNA and DNA product (through the protein coat of the virus), which allows for the succession of affinity selection and amplification of selected phage particles resulting in powerful enrichment of selected phage and an increase in assay sensitivity [160;161]. This link between *genotype* and *phenotype* is absent in lambda phage expression library screening assays used to identify ligands for different targets [162;163]. These assays are more labour-intensive and are characterized by lower sensitivities due to the preclusion of phage enrichment.

A commonly used phage display procedure encompasses the display of synthetically produced peptide libraries [164]. This peptide phage display technique has already been applied by several research groups for autoantibody profiling in MS and RA.

The peptide phage display technique was applied by Cortese *et al.* to identify peptide motifs that were recognized by antibodies in the CSF from MS patients. The authors showed that selection with individual MS CSF led to the identification of patient-specific epitopes. Moreover, antibodies against the selected epitopes were demonstrated with a similar frequency in MS sera as compared to control sera [165]. In a new attempt to identify MS-specific epitopes, 20 different MS CSF samples were pooled for selection of a random peptide library, confirming the earlier finding of patient-specific antibody reactivities. The authors concluded that common antibody specificities are absent in MS patients, or that they are present in very low concentrations [166].

However, other research groups who adopted similar peptide phage display strategies for autoantibody profiling in MS were successful at identifying MS-associated peptide motifs. A similar peptide phage display approach was applied by Dybwad *et al.*, who analyzed the CSF antibody specificities within an oligoclonal band from one MS patient using different phage displayed random peptide libraries. Distinct but structurally related peptide motifs were detected, which showed significant linear homology with collagen proteins, the 68 kDa neurofilament protein, versican and other proteins from viruses such as human cytomegalovirus, herpes simplex virus and human papillomavirus [167].

Jolivet-Reynaud *et al.* reported the use of a decapeptide phage display library to analyze the antibody specificities in the CSF and serum from 4 MS patients. The peptides that were identified by selections with MS serum were not disease-specific while selections performed with CSF resulted in the identification of several motifs which were recognized more specifically in MS CSF compared to CSF from patients with other neurological diseases. Amino acid similarities were detected between the selected peptides and envelope regions of MS-associated retrovirus and the related endogenous retrovirus (HERV-W) [168].

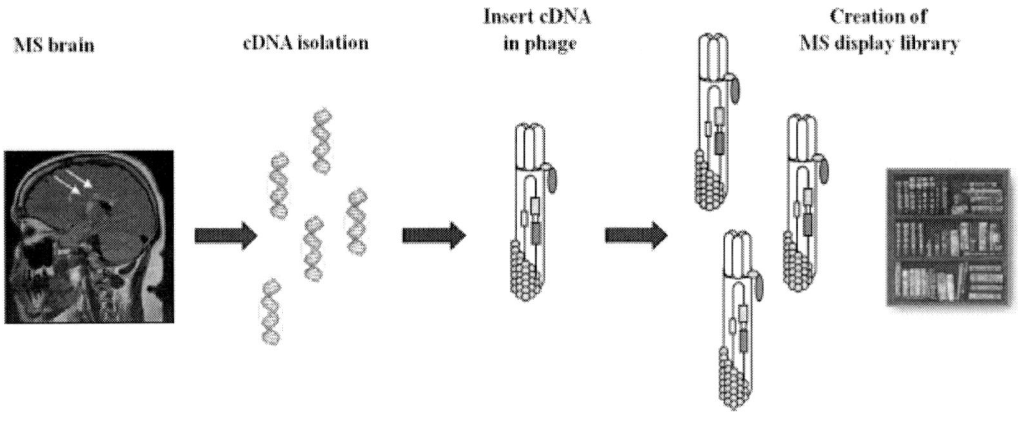

Figure 2. Creation of a cDNA phage display library. The antigenic complexity of diseased tissue is far greater than that of normal tissue. Therefore, MS brain plaques with varying degrees of demyelination and inflammatory activity are used for the construction of the MS cDNA phage display library. cDNA from the MS plaques is isolated and subsequently incorporated in the genome of filamentous bacteriophages. Upon phage virion assembly, the (poly)peptide product, encoded by the inserted cDNA, will be expressed at the phage surface as a fusion product with the phage coat protein. By inserting multiple cDNA products in phages, a diverse cDNA library is created.

Rand *et al.* have used individual CSF from 14 MS patients for the screening of a hexamer peptide phage display library. A common motif was selected, which was found in EBV protein EBNA1, alpha B crystalline and in the 65 kDa non-structural cytomegalovirus antigen. It was shown that 60-65% of EBV-seropositive MS patients presented with antibodies against the selected motif [169;170].

The main drawback of the peptide phage display approach is the identification of so-called mimotopes [171]. Mimotopes are peptides forming epitopes that structurally mimic the actual *in vivo* antigens. This implies that the mimotope and the corresponding actual antigen are not necessarily identical or similar at amino acid level, although sequence similarity is not excluded. The identification of the actual *in vivo* antigen of the detected autoantibody requires a labour-intensive and difficult characterization of the identified epitope [172]. This drawback of peptide phage display can partially be overcome by application of cDNA phage display [173]. cDNA phage display entails the display of an entire cDNA expression library allowing interaction between cDNA encoded peptides and proteins exposed on the surface of the phage and antibody selectors. An expression library can be conveniently constructed from cell lines and cell cultures. cDNA phage display of an expression library made from diseased target tissue is even more interesting. The use of affected tissue allows the display of the entire heterogeneous antigen composition within the diseased tissue.

We have developed and used a powerful molecular multiplexing procedure called serological antigen selection (SAS) of which the strength lies within the application of cDNA phage display. Application of the procedure for MS CSF entailed filamentous phage display of a normalized expression library made from three active chronic MS plaques with varying degrees of demyelination and inflammatory activity, obtained from one MS patient (Fig. 2) [174]. By using a cDNA expression library from diseased tissue for phage display library construction, the entire heterogeneity of known and novel expressed antigens present within the affected tissue can be displayed and potentially selected. The antigenic complexity held within the diseased tissue is far greater than that from normal tissue, due to the diversity of processes occurring at this site of autoimmune attack such as inflammatory cell infiltration, activation and migration as well as destruction and possible repair of endogenous tissue cells. Sequencing of the MS cDNA library confirmed the value of the use of a cDNA expression library made from diseased tissue for the identification of autoantibody targets in MS [175]. The percentage of novel genes and the number of expressed sequences were significantly higher in the MS library compared to normal human brain libraries. The detected sequences were associated with the diversity of processes occurring in and around MS lesions such as inflammatory cell infiltration, activation and migration, antigen presentation and tissue damage [176]. By application of affinity selections on the MS cDNA phage display library with pooled CSF from 10 RRMS patients, we recently identified a panel of 4 MS-specific and 4 MS-associated antigenic targets [177]. Immunoreactivity against this panel of 8 novel MS-candidate antigens was analyzed in 73 MS patients, 64 patients with non-inflammatory neurological diseases and 30 patients with other inflammatory neurological diseases. The sensitivity and specificity values of the detection of antibodies against this panel of 8 autoantibody targets for MS were 45% and 86%, respectively [178]. Further research is needed to evaluate the biological role of these antigenic targets in the disease process of MS.

5.2. B Cell Reactivity Analysis in MS

Instead of focusing on autoantibody profiling, some studies have analyzed the reactivity of the clonally expanded B cells and plasma cells in the CSF and/or peripheral blood of MS patients. The group of Link *et al.* performed different studies on B cell reactivity in MS using an immunospot assay. Nitrocellulose microtiter plates were coated with myelin antigens to detect binding of peripheral blood mononuclear cells (PBMC) or CSF cells. When studying CSF cells and PBMC of 19 MS patients, MBP-reactive CSF B cells were found in 57% of MS patients while none were present in peripheral blood. MAG-reactive B cells were indicated both in CSF and PBMC of MS patients (55% and 11% of patients, respectively) [179]. Furthermore, anti-MOG IgG secreting cells were demonstrated in PBMC from 8 of 16 MS patients and in CSF from 8 of 10 MS patients [180].

Other studies made use of recombinant antibodies that were produced from patients' B cells. $CD19^+$ or $CD138^+$ cells from CSF were single-cell sorted into PCR plates, the variable regions of the heavy and light Ig chains (V_H and V_L) were amplified and cloned into a plasmid vector which was then expressed in a bacterial expression system. The corresponding recombinant antibodies were used for reactivity screenings with immunoprecipitation, Western blot, ELISA or immunohistochemistry. Lambracht-Washington and coworkers discovered reactivity of their recombinantly produced antibodies towards MBP, 2',3'-cyclic nucleotide 3'-phosphodiesterase (CNPase) and GFAP [181]. On the other hand, von Büdingen *et al.* produced 9 recombinant MS antibodies following the same procedure, and in this case 8 displayed myelin reactivity and 1 was directed against astroglia [182]. Apart from myelin binding in MS brain tissue, their targets could not be identified using several techniques such as costaining with known myelin antigens on brain tissue in immunohistochemistry, Western blot with human myelin or ELISA using recombinant and native MOG and MBP. In yet another study from Zhang *et al.*, recombinant antibodies from MS CSF demonstrated reactivity to axons with pathologic changes in MS brain tissue [183]. The targets were later identified as TPI and GAPDH [184]. Very recently, Yu *et al.* employed 19 recombinant antibodies from clonally expanded plasma cells in the CSF of MS patients in combination with phage displayed random peptide libraries to demonstrate peptide reactivity [185]. Several antigenic candidates were identified, including stress proteins, cell surface proteins and neuronal proteins.

Another possibility for determination of the B cell target antigens and characterization of the B cell repertoire is the immortalization of B cells from MS patients. Using this technique immortalized B cell clones, that show continuous antibody production, are generated. The target antigens of the produced antibodies can be determined and the B cell response that is going on in vivo can be studied.

5.2.1. B Cell Immortalization

B cell immortalization by EBV has been widely used in immunological, molecular and genetic research as it provides high amounts of DNA and large numbers of B cells and antibody molecules. EBV infects B cells via their CD21 receptor [186] and subsequently transforms them into continually dividing, lymphoblastoid cell lines. Its advantage over other monoclonal antibody producing technologies is the generation of antibodies that represent both the specificity and diversity of the humoral immune response in vivo. Consequently, antibodies produced by B cell immortalization can be useful in several settings in which humoral immunity is involved. Antibodies can even be generated against an infectious agent or tumour cells, rendering these antibodies attractive for therapy.

In vitro infection of B cells from human peripheral blood by EBV causes a transformation into actively proliferating lymphoblastoid cell lines (LCL) [187]. The continuous proliferation of these LCL may be the consequence of the absence of a GC environment where EBNA2, 3A, 3B, 3C and LP are normally downregulated [188]. Shortening of the telomeres occurs because of fast cell division, until the transformed cells go into a proliferative crisis [189]. At this point little or no telomeric DNA remains, leading to apoptosis of a large proportion of the LCL [190]. A small proportion of the transformed cells survive the proliferative crisis through activation of telomerase, the enzyme that elongates telomeres de novo (Fig. 3) [191-193]. They become truly immortalized B cell lines that are characterized by downregulation of p16/Rb [187], mutation of the p53 gene [194], modulation of apoptosis [190], upregulation of WRN helicase [194;195], chromosomal instability [194] and a change in cytotoxicity to various chemical compounds [196]. All these features contribute to the evasion of cell death and continuous cell growth.

We have developed an improved B cell immortalization method that is characterized by immortalization efficiencies up to 83% for the generation of IgG-producing immortalized B cell lines from the peripheral blood [197]. Moreover, almost 90% of the produced immortalized B cell lines appeared to be monoclonal, which eliminated the need for subcloning. For the first time, a B cell immortalization procedure was introduced with high efficiency and reproducibility for low B cell numbers that made immediate generation of monoclonal antibodies, representing the in vivo humoral immune response, possible.

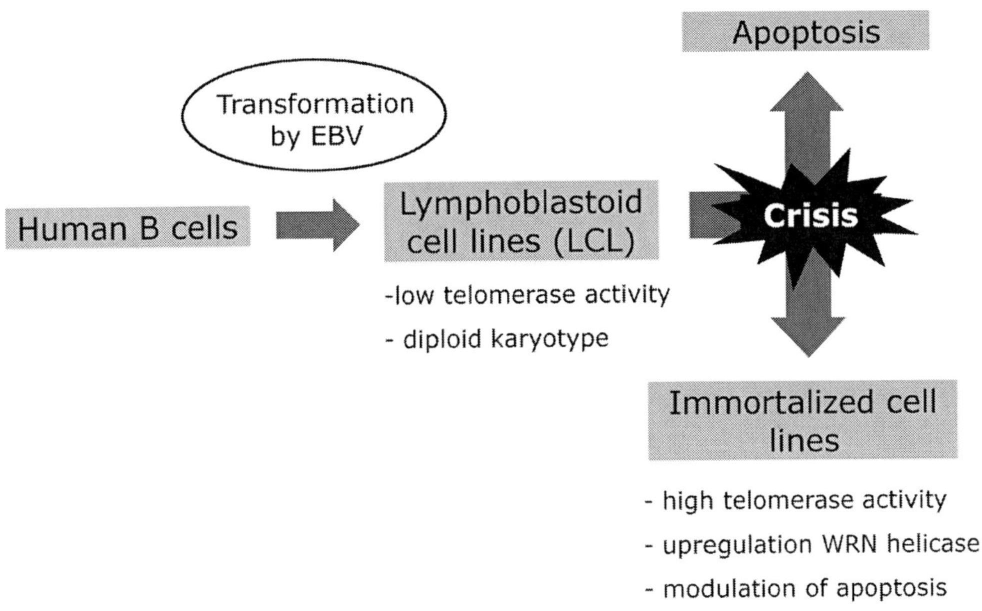

Figure 3. In vitro B cell immortalization process. Human B cells can become infected by EBV and will be transformed into lymphoblastoid cell lines (LCL), characterized by low telomerase activity and normal diploid karyotypes. When telomeres are very short, the transformed B cells go into a proliferative crisis in which most of the cells die because of apoptosis. A small portion of the B cells survive and become immortalized through activation of telomerase. Some other features of immortalized B cells are the upregulation of WRN helicase and modulation of apoptosis.

5.2.2. Application of B Cell Immortalization in MS Reactivity Profiling

Using this optimized B cell immortalization method, we have already been able to produce a large panel of immortalized B cell lines from the peripheral blood of MS patients and CIS patients that experienced a first clinical manifestation of MS-like disease [198;199]. Some B cell lines could also be recovered from the CSF of a MS patient. Intracellular autoreactivity of a proportion of the generated immortalized B cell lines from the peripheral blood was demonstrated by analysis of antibody binding to a human oligodendroglioma (HOG) cell line, PBMC and a control human alveolar epithelial (A549) cell line. Further, the immortalized cultures were successfully used for molecular analysis of the Ig heavy chain genes of peripheral and intrathecal B cells. A restricted antigen-stimulated clonally expanded B cell response with possible affinity maturation was hereby demonstrated, not only in CSF but also in peripheral blood of MS and CIS patients (unpublished results). In addition, autoreactivity against striated muscle proteins was shown for immortalized B cell lines that were recovered from MG patients using the same immortalization procedure [200].

These data show how autoreactive antibodies can be produced from patients with autoimmune disease using B cell immortalization. Characterization of these antibodies and identification of the target antigens of these clonally expanded B cells could provide more insight into their relevance in the disease process but could also lead to the identification of novel antigenic targets in MS.

6. Conclusion

Due to the preliminary positive effect of B cell depletion therapy in MS patients, there is renewed interest in the role of autoreactive B cells and autoantibodies in the disease process of multiple sclerosis. Reactivity analysis of the humoral immune response through investigation of autoantibody profiles and B cell reactivity resulted in the identification of a wide range of different B cell and autoantibody targets in MS patients.

However, despite the advances in the knowledge on the humoral reactivity profile in MS patients, up till now, not one autoreactivity was specifically associated with MS. Also, none of the detected autoreactivities was detected in all MS patients. These findings point towards the presence of different autoreactivity profiles in different MS patients, exemplified by the characteristic heterogeneity of the disease. The use of new, highly sensitive and preferably multiplexing technologies such as SAS and EBV B cell immortalization in reactivity analysis can be valuable to expand our current knowledge on the humoral reactivity profile in MS patients.

The elucidation of the MS-associated autoreactivity profile is valuable from a diagnostic biomarker point of view. In addition, the discovery of novel targets of the humoral autoimmune response in MS patients will generate valuable knowledge regarding underlying disease processes and etiology of MS, and can lead to the identification of highly needed, novel therapeutic targets.

7. References

[1] Traugott U, Reinherz EL, Raine CS. Multiple sclerosis. Distribution of T cells, T cell subsets and Ia-positive macrophages in lesions of different ages. *J Neuroimmunol* 1983; 4(3):201-221.

[2] Zamvil SS, Steinman L. The T lymphocyte in experimental allergic encephalomyelitis. *Annu Rev Immunol* 1990; 8:579-621.

[3] Bar-Or A, Calabresi PA, Arnold D, Markowitz C, Shafer S, Kasper LH, Waubant E, Gazda S, Fox RJ, Panzara M, Sarkar N, Agarwal S, Smith CH. Rituximab in relapsing-remitting multiple sclerosis: a 72-week, open-label, phase I trial. *Ann Neurol* 2008; 63(3):395-400.

[4] Stuve O, Leussink VI, Frohlich R, Hemmer B, Hartung HP, Menge T, Kieseier BC. Long-term B-lymphocyte depletion with rituximab in patients with relapsing-remitting multiple sclerosis. *Arch Neurol* 2009; 66(2):259-261.

[5] Naismith RT, Piccio L, Lyons JA, Lauber J, Tutlam NT, Parks BJ, Trinkaus K, Song SK, Cross AH. Rituximab add-on therapy for breakthrough relapsing multiple sclerosis: a 52-week phase II trial. *Neurology* 2010; 74(23):1860-1867.

[6] Hauser SL, Waubant E, Arnold DL, Vollmer T, Antel J, Fox RJ, Bar-Or A, Panzara M, Sarkar N, Agarwal S, Langer-Gould A, Smith CH. B-cell depletion with rituximab in relapsing-remitting multiple sclerosis. *N Engl J Med* 2008; 358(7):676-688.

[7] Klein U, Rajewsky K, Kuppers R. Human immunoglobulin (Ig)M+IgD+ peripheral blood B cells expressing the CD27 cell surface antigen carry somatically mutated variable region genes: CD27 as a general marker for somatically mutated (memory) B cells. *J Exp Med* 1998; 188(9):1679-1689.

[8] Blink EJ, Light A, Kallies A, Nutt SL, Hodgkin PD, Tarlinton DM. Early appearance of germinal center-derived memory B cells and plasma cells in blood after primary immunization. *J Exp Med* 2005; 201(4):545-554.

[9] Loken MR, Shah VO, Dattilio KL, Civin CI. Flow cytometric analysis of human bone marrow. II. Normal B lymphocyte development. *Blood* 1987; 70(5):1316-1324.

[10] Ochsenbein AF, Pinschewer DD, Sierro S, Horvath E, Hengartner H, Zinkernagel RM. Protective long-term antibody memory by antigen-driven and T help-dependent differentiation of long-lived memory B cells to short-lived plasma cells independent of secondary lymphoid organs. *Proc Natl Acad Sci* U S A 2000; 97(24):13263-13268.

[11] Klein U, Tu Y, Stolovitzky GA, Keller JL, Haddad J, Jr., Miljkovic V, Cattoretti G, Califano A, Dalla-Favera R. Transcriptional analysis of the B cell germinal center reaction. *Proc Natl Acad Sci* U S A 2003; 100(5):2639-2644.

[12] Dorner T, Radbruch A. Selecting B cells and plasma cells to memory. *J Exp Med* 2005; 201(4):497-499.

[13] Berek C, Berger A, Apel M. Maturation of the immune response in germinal centers. *Cell* 1991; 67(6):1121-1129.

[14] MacLennan IC. Germinal centers. *Annu Rev Immunol* 1994; 12:117-139.

[15] Le Pottier L, Devauchelle V, Pers JO, Jamin C, Youinou P. The mosaic of B-cell subsets (with special emphasis on primary Sjogren's syndrome). *Autoimmun Rev* 2007; 6(3):149-154.

[16] Meinl E, Krumbholz M, Hohlfeld R. B lineage cells in the inflammatory central nervous system environment: migration, maintenance, local antibody production, and therapeutic modulation. *Ann Neurol* 2006; 59(6):880-892.

[17] Cepok S, Rosche B, Grummel V, Vogel F, Zhou D, Sayn J, Sommer N, Hartung HP, Hemmer B. Short-lived plasma blasts are the main B cell effector subset during the course of multiple sclerosis. *Brain* 2005; 128(Pt 7):1667-1676.

[18] Corcione A, Casazza S, Ferretti E, Giunti D, Zappia E, Pistorio A, Gambini C, Mancardi GL, Uccelli A, Pistoia V. Recapitulation of B cell differentiation in the central nervous system of patients with multiple sclerosis. *Proc Natl Acad Sci* U S A 2004; 101(30):11064-11069.

[19] Corcione A, Aloisi F, Serafini B, Capello E, Mancardi GL, Pistoia V, Uccelli A. B-cell differentiation in the CNS of patients with multiple sclerosis. *Autoimmun Rev* 2005; 4(8):549-554.

[20] Kuenz B, Lutterotti A, Ehling R, Gneiss C, Haemmerle M, Rainer C, Deisenhammer F, Schocke M, Berger T, Reindl M. Cerebrospinal fluid B cells correlate with early brain inflammation in multiple sclerosis. *PLoS ONE* 2008; 3(7):e2559.

[21] Ritchie AM, Gilden DH, Williamson RA, Burgoon MP, Yu X, Helm K, Corboy JR, Owens GP. Comparative analysis of the CD19+ and CD138+ cell antibody repertoires in the cerebrospinal fluid of patients with multiple sclerosis. J Immunol 2004; 173(1):649-656.

[22] Cepok S, von Geldern G, Grummel V, Hochgesand S, Celik H, Hartung H, Hemmer B. Accumulation of class switched IgD-IgM- memory B cells in the cerebrospinal fluid during neuroinflammation. *J Neuroimmunol* 2006; 180(1-2):33-39.

[23] Pascual V, Liu YJ, Magalski A, de Bouteiller O, Banchereau J, Capra JD. Analysis of somatic mutation in five B cell subsets of human tonsil. *J Exp Med* 1994; 180(1):329-339.

[24] Serafini B, Rosicarelli B, Magliozzi R, Stigliano E, Aloisi F. Detection of ectopic B-cell follicles with germinal centers in the meninges of patients with secondary progressive multiple sclerosis. *Brain Pathol* 2004; 14(2):164-174.

[25] Winges KM, Gilden DH, Bennett JL, Yu X, Ritchie AM, Owens GP. Analysis of multiple sclerosis cerebrospinal fluid reveals a continuum of clonally related antibody-secreting cells that are predominantly plasma blasts. *J Neuroimmunol* 2007; 192(1-2):226-234.

[26] Jego G, Robillard N, Puthier D, Amiot M, Accard F, Pineau D, Harousseau JL, Bataille R, Pellat-Deceunynck C. Reactive plasmacytoses are expansions of plasmablasts retaining the capacity to differentiate into plasma cells. *Blood* 1999; 94(2):701-712.

[27] Archelos JJ, Storch MK, Hartung HP. The role of B cells and autoantibodies in multiple sclerosis. *Ann Neurol* 2000; 47(6):694-706.

[28] Cepok S, Jacobsen M, Schock S, Omer B, Jaekel S, Boddeker I, Oertel WH, Sommer N, Hemmer B. Patterns of cerebrospinal fluid pathology correlate with disease progression in multiple sclerosis. *Brain* 2001; 124(Pt 11):2169-2176.

[29] Cross AH, Trotter JL, Lyons J. B cells and antibodies in CNS demyelinating disease. J Neuroimmunol 2001; 112(1-2):1-14.

[30] Dalakas MC. B cells as therapeutic targets in autoimmune neurological disorders. *Nat Clin Pract Neurol* 2008; 4(10):557-567.

[31] Qin Y, Duquette P. B-cell immunity in MS. *Int MS J* 2003; 10(4):110-120.

[32] Bhakdi S, Tranum-Jensen J. Complement lysis: a hole is a hole. *Immunol Today* 1991; 12(9):318-320.
[33] Duddy ME, Alter A, Bar-Or A. Distinct profiles of human B cell effector cytokines: a role in immune regulation? *J Immunol* 2004; 172(6):3422-3427.
[34] Ziemssen T, Ziemssen F. The role of the humoral immune system in multiple sclerosis (MS) and its animal model experimental autoimmune encephalomyelitis (EAE). *Autoimmun Rev* 2005; 4(7):460-467.
[35] Lanzavecchia A. Receptor-mediated antigen uptake and its effect on antigen presentation to class II-restricted T lymphocytes. *Annu Rev Immunol* 1990; 8:773-793.
[36] Rock KL, Benacerraf B, Abbas AK. Antigen presentation by hapten-specific B lymphocytes. I. Role of surface immunoglobulin receptors. *J Exp Med* 1984; 160(4):1102-1113.
[37] Genc K, Dona DL, Reder AT. Increased CD80(+) B cells in active multiple sclerosis and reversal by interferon beta-1b therapy. *J Clin Invest* 1997; 99(11):2664-2671.
[38] Niino M, Hirotani M, Miyazaki Y, Sasaki H. Memory and naive B-cell subsets in patients with multiple sclerosis. *Neurosci Lett* 2009; 464(1):74-78.
[39] Torcia M, Bracci-Laudiero L, Lucibello M, Nencioni L, Labardi D, Rubartelli A, Cozzolino F, Aloe L, Garaci E. Nerve growth factor is an autocrine survival factor for memory B lymphocytes. *Cell* 1996; 85(3):345-356.
[40] Kerschensteiner M, Gallmeier E, Behrens L, Leal VV, Misgeld T, Klinkert WE, Kolbeck R, Hoppe E, Oropeza-Wekerle RL, Bartke I, Stadelmann C, Lassmann H, Wekerle H, Hohlfeld R. Activated human T cells, B cells, and monocytes produce brain-derived neurotrophic factor in vitro and in inflammatory brain lesions: a neuroprotective role of inflammation? *J Exp Med* 1999; 189(5):865-870.
[41] Vargas-Leal V, Bruno R, Derfuss T, Krumbholz M, Hohlfeld R, Meinl E. Expression and function of glial cell line-derived neurotrophic factor family ligands and their receptors on human immune cells. *J Immunol* 2005; 175(4):2301-2308.
[42] Alter A, Duddy M, Hebert S, Biernacki K, Prat A, Antel JP, Yong VW, Nuttall RK, Pennington CJ, Edwards DR, Bar-Or A. Determinants of human B cell migration across brain endothelial cells. *J Immunol* 2003; 170(9):4497-4505.
[43] Krumbholz M, Theil D, Cepok S, Hemmer B, Kivisakk P, Ransohoff RM, Hofbauer M, Farina C, Derfuss T, Hartle C, Newcombe J, Hohlfeld R, Meinl E. Chemokines in multiple sclerosis: CXCL12 and CXCL13 up-regulation is differentially linked to CNS immune cell recruitment. *Brain* 2006; 129(Pt 1):200-211.
[44] Avery DT, Kalled SL, Ellyard JI, Ambrose C, Bixler SA, Thien M, Brink R, Mackay F, Hodgkin PD, Tangye SG. BAFF selectively enhances the survival of plasmablasts generated from human memory B cells. *J Clin Invest* 2003; 112(2):286-297.
[45] Schneider P. The role of APRIL and BAFF in lymphocyte activation. *Curr Opin Immunol* 2005; 17(3):282-289.
[46] Meinl E, Derfuss T, Krumbholz M, Probstel AK, Hohlfeld R. Humoral autoimmunity in multiple sclerosis. *J Neurol Sci* 2010.
[47] Krumbholz M, Theil D, Derfuss T, Rosenwald A, Schrader F, Monoranu CM, Kalled SL, Hess DM, Serafini B, Aloisi F, Wekerle H, Hohlfeld R, Meinl E. BAFF is produced by astrocytes and up-regulated in multiple sclerosis lesions and primary central nervous system lymphoma. *J Exp Med* 2005; 201(2):195-200.

[48] Thangarajh M, Gomes A, Masterman T, Hillert J, Hjelmstrom P. Expression of B-cell-activating factor of the TNF family (BAFF) and its receptors in multiple sclerosis. *J Neuroimmunol* 2004; 152(1-2):183-190.

[49] Thangarajh M, Masterman T, Rot U, Duvefelt K, Brynedal B, Karrenbauer VD, Hillert J. Increased levels of APRIL (a proliferation-inducing ligand) mRNA in multiple sclerosis. *J Neuroimmunol* 2005; 167(1-2):210-214.

[50] Serafini B, Rosicarelli B, Franciotta D, Magliozzi R, Reynolds R, Cinque P, Andreoni L, Trivedi P, Salvetti M, Faggioni A, Aloisi F. Dysregulated Epstein-Barr virus infection in the multiple sclerosis brain. *J Exp Med* 2007; 204(12):2899-2912.

[51] Daridon C, Youinou P, Pers JO. BAFF, APRIL, TWE-PRIL: who's who? *Autoimmun Rev* 2008; 7(4):267-271.

[52] Laterre EC, Callewaert A, Heremans JF, Sfaello Z. Electrophoretic morphology of gamma globulins in cerebrospinal fluid of multiple sclerosis and other diseases of the nervous system. *Neurology* 1970; 20(10):982-990.

[53] Kabat EA, Glusman M, Knaub V. Quantitative estimation of the albumin and gamma-globulin in normal and pathological cerebrospinal fluid by immunochemical methods. *Am J Med* 1948; 4:653-662.

[54] Irani D. Cerebrospinal fluid. In *Clinical Practice.* Philadelphia, USA: Saunders Elsevier, 2009.

[55] Walsh MJ, Tourtellotte WW. Temporal invariance and clonal uniformity of brain and cerebrospinal IgG, IgA, and IgM in multiple sclerosis. *J Exp Med* 1986; 163(1):41-53.

[56] Walsh MJ, Tourtellotte WW. Temporal invariance and clonal uniformity of brain and cerebrospinal IgG, IgA, and IgM in multiple sclerosis. *J Exp Med* 1986; 163(1):41-53.

[57] Freedman MS, Thompson EJ, Deisenhammer F, Giovannoni G, Grimsley G, Keir G, Ohman S, Racke MK, Sharief M, Sindic CJ, Sellebjerg F, Tourtellotte WW. Recommended standard of cerebrospinal fluid analysis in the diagnosis of multiple sclerosis: a consensus statement. *Arch Neurol* 2005; 62(6):865-870.

[58] McDonald WI, Compston A, Edan G, Goodkin D, Hartung HP, Lublin FD, McFarland HF, Paty DW, Polman CH, Reingold SC, Sandberg-Wollheim M, Sibley W, Thompson A, Van Den NS, Weinshenker BY, Wolinsky JS. Recommended diagnostic criteria for multiple sclerosis: guidelines from the International Panel on the diagnosis of multiple sclerosis. *Ann Neurol* 2001; 50(1):121-127.

[59] Qin Y, Duquette P, Zhang Y, Olek M, Da RR, Richardson J, Antel JP, Talbot P, Cashman NR, Tourtellotte WW, Wekerle H, Van Den NS. Intrathecal B-cell clonal expansion, an early sign of humoral immunity, in the cerebrospinal fluid of patients with clinically isolated syndrome suggestive of multiple sclerosis. *Lab Invest* 2003; 83(7):1081-1088.

[60] Baranzini SE, Jeong MC, Butunoi C, Murray RS, Bernard CC, Oksenberg JR. B cell repertoire diversity and clonal expansion in multiple sclerosis brain lesions. *J Immunol* 1999; 163(9):5133-5144.

[61] Cepok S, Rosche B, Grummel V, Vogel F, Zhou D, Sayn J, Sommer N, Hartung HP, Hemmer B. Short-lived plasma blasts are the main B cell effector subset during the course of multiple sclerosis. *Brain* 2005; 128(Pt 7):1667-1676.

[62] Genain CP, Cannella B, Hauser SL, Raine CS. Identification of autoantibodies associated with myelin damage in multiple sclerosis. *Nat Med* 1999; 5(2):170-175.

[63] Lassmann H, Bruck W, Lucchinetti C. Heterogeneity of multiple sclerosis pathogenesis: implications for diagnosis and therapy. *Trends Mol Med* 2001; 7(3):115-121.

[64] Cross AH, Trotter JL, Lyons J. B cells and antibodies in CNS demyelinating disease. *J Neuroimmunol* 2001; 112(1-2):1-14.

[65] Lucchinetti C, Bruck W, Parisi J, Scheithauer B, Rodriguez M, Lassmann H. Heterogeneity of multiple sclerosis lesions: implications for the pathogenesis of demyelination. *Ann Neurol* 2000; 47(6):707-717.

[66] Serafini B, Rosicarelli B, Magliozzi R, Stigliano E, Aloisi F. Detection of ectopic B-cell follicles with germinal centers in the meninges of patients with secondary progressive multiple sclerosis. *Brain Pathol* 2004; 14(2):164-174.

[67] Corcione A, Aloisi F, Serafini B, Capello E, Mancardi GL, Pistoia V, Uccelli A. B-cell differentiation in the CNS of patients with multiple sclerosis. *Autoimmun Rev* 2005; 4(8):549-554.

[68] Aloisi F, Serafini B, Magliozzi R, Howell OW, Reynolds R. *Detection of Epstein-Barr virus and B-cell follicles in the multiple sclerosis brain: what you find depends on how and where you look.* Brain 2010.

[69] Magliozzi R, Columba-Cabezas S, Serafini B, Aloisi F. Intracerebral expression of CXCL13 and BAFF is accompanied by formation of lymphoid follicle-like structures in the meninges of mice with relapsing experimental autoimmune encephalomyelitis. *J Neuroimmunol* 2004; 148(1-2):11-23.

[70] Izquierdo G, Angulo S, Garcia-Moreno JM, Gamero MA, Navarro G, Gata JM, Ruiz-Pena JL, Paramo MD. Intrathecal IgG synthesis: marker of progression in multiple sclerosis patients. *Acta Neurol Scand* 2002; 105(3):158-163.

[71] Linington C, Bradl M, Lassmann H, Brunner C, Vass K. Augmentation of demyelination in rat acute allergic encephalomyelitis by circulating mouse monoclonal antibodies directed against a myelin/oligodendrocyte glycoprotein. *Am J Pathol* 1988; 130(3):443-454.

[72] Morris-Downes MM, Smith PA, Rundle JL, Piddlesden SJ, Baker D, Pham-Dinh D, Heijmans N, Amor S. Pathological and regulatory effects of anti-myelin antibodies in experimental allergic encephalomyelitis in mice. *J Neuroimmunol* 2002; 125(1-2):114-124.

[73] Mathey EK, Derfuss T, Storch MK, Williams KR, Hales K, Woolley DR, Al Hayani A, Davies SN, Rasband MN, Olsson T, Moldenhauer A, Velhin S, Hohlfeld R, Meinl E, Linington C. Neurofascin as a novel target for autoantibody-mediated axonal injury. *J Exp Med* 2007; 204(10):2363-2372.

[74] Martin MP, Monson NL. Potential role of humoral immunity in the pathogenesis of multiple sclerosis (MS) and experimental autoimmune encephalomyelitis (EAE). *Front Biosci* 2007; 12:2735-2749.

[75] Keegan M, Konig F, McClelland R, Bruck W, Morales Y, Bitsch A, Panitch H, Lassmann H, Weinshenker B, Rodriguez M, Parisi J, Lucchinetti CF. Relation between humoral pathological changes in multiple sclerosis and response to therapeutic plasma exchange. *Lancet* 2005; 366(9485):579-582.

[76] Cross AH, Stark JL, Lauber J, Ramsbottom MJ, Lyons JA. Rituximab reduces B cells and T cells in cerebrospinal fluid of multiple sclerosis patients. *J Neuroimmunol* 2006; 180(1-2):63-70.

[77] Hauser SL, Waubant E, Arnold DL, Vollmer T, Antel J, Fox RJ, Bar-Or A, Panzara M, Sarkar N, Agarwal S, Langer-Gould A, Smith CH. B-cell depletion with rituximab in relapsing-remitting multiple sclerosis. *N Engl J Med* 2008; 358(7):676-688.

[78] Kerschensteiner M, Gallmeier E, Behrens L, Leal VV, Misgeld T, Klinkert WE, Kolbeck R, Hoppe E, Oropeza-Wekerle RL, Bartke I, Stadelmann C, Lassmann H, Wekerle H, Hohlfeld R. Activated human T cells, B cells, and monocytes produce brain-derived neurotrophic factor in vitro and in inflammatory brain lesions: a neuroprotective role of inflammation? *J Exp Med* 1999; 189(5):865-870.

[79] Fillatreau S, Sweenie CH, McGeachy MJ, Gray D, Anderton SM. B cells regulate autoimmunity by provision of IL-10. *Nat Immunol* 2002; 3(10):944-950.

[80] Warrington AE, Asakura K, Bieber AJ, Ciric B, Van K, V, Kaveri SV, Kyle RA, Pease LR, Rodriguez M. Human monoclonal antibodies reactive to oligodendrocytes promote remyelination in a model of multiple sclerosis. *Proc Natl Acad Sci* U S A 2000; 97(12):6820-6825.

[81] Cross AH, Trotter JL, Lyons J. B cells and antibodies in CNS demyelinating disease. *J Neuroimmunol* 2001; 112(1-2):1-14.

[82] Cepok S, Zhou D, Srivastava R, Nessler S, Stei S, Bussow K, Sommer N, Hemmer B. Identification of Epstein-Barr virus proteins as putative targets of the immune response in multiple sclerosis. *J Clin Invest* 2005; 115(5):1352-1360.

[83] Quintana FJ, Farez MF, Viglietta V, Iglesias AH, Merbl Y, Izquierdo G, Lucas M, Basso AS, Khoury SJ, Lucchinetti CF, Cohen IR, Weiner HL. Antigen microarrays identify unique serum autoantibody signatures in clinical and pathologic subtypes of multiple sclerosis. *Proc Natl Acad Sci* U S A 2008; 105(48):18889-18894.

[84] Zhou D, Srivastava R, Nessler S, Grummel V, Sommer N, Bruck W, Hartung HP, Stadelmann C, Hemmer B. Identification of a pathogenic antibody response to native myelin oligodendrocyte glycoprotein in multiple sclerosis. *Proc Natl Acad Sci* U S A 2006; 103(50):19057-19062.

[85] Reindl M, Khalil M, Berger T. Antibodies as biological markers for pathophysiological processes in MS. *J Neuroimmunol* 2006; 180(1-2):50-62.

[86] Huizinga R, Linington C, Amor S. Resistance is futile: antineuronal autoimmunity in multiple sclerosis. *Trends Immunol* 2008; 29(2):54-60.

[87] Reindl M, Linington C, Brehm U, Egg R, Dilitz E, Deisenhammer F, Poewe W, Berger T. Antibodies against the myelin oligodendrocyte glycoprotein and the myelin basic protein in multiple sclerosis and other neurological diseases: a comparative study. *Brain* 1999; 122 (Pt 11):2047-2056.

[88] Reindl M, Linington C, Brehm U, Egg R, Dilitz E, Deisenhammer F, Poewe W, Berger T. Antibodies against the myelin oligodendrocyte glycoprotein and the myelin basic protein in multiple sclerosis and other neurological diseases: a comparative study. *Brain* 1999; 122 (Pt 11):2047-2056.

[89] Sun JB, Olsson T, Wang WZ, Xiao BG, Kostulas V, Fredrikson S, Ekre HP, Link H. Autoreactive T and B cells responding to myelin proteolipid protein in multiple sclerosis and controls. *Eur J Immunol* 1991; 21(6):1461-1468.

[90] Moller JR, Johnson D, Brady RO, Tourtellotte WW, Quarles RH. Antibodies to myelin-associated glycoprotein (MAG) in the cerebrospinal fluid of multiple sclerosis patients. *J Neuroimmunol* 1989; 22(1):55-61.

[91] O'Connor KC, Chitnis T, Griffin DE, Piyasirisilp S, Bar-Or A, Khoury S, Wucherpfennig KW, Hafler DA. Myelin basic protein-reactive autoantibodies in the serum and cerebrospinal fluid of multiple sclerosis patients are characterized by low-affinity interactions. *J Neuroimmunol* 2003; 136(1-2):140-148.
[92] Pittock SJ, Reindl M, Achenbach S, Berger T, Bruck W, Konig F, Morales Y, Lassmann H, Bryant S, Moore SB, Keegan BM, Lucchinetti CF. Myelin oligodendrocyte glycoprotein antibodies in pathologically proven multiple sclerosis: frequency, stability and clinicopathologic correlations. *Mult Scler* 2007; 13(1):7-16.
[93] Lim ET, Berger T, Reindl M, Dalton CM, Fernando K, Keir G, Thompson EJ, Miller DH, Giovannoni G. Anti-myelin antibodies do not allow earlier diagnosis of multiple sclerosis. *Mult Scler* 2005; 11(4):492-494.
[94] Reindl M, Linington C, Brehm U, Egg R, Dilitz E, Deisenhammer F, Poewe W, Berger T. Antibodies against the myelin oligodendrocyte glycoprotein and the myelin basic protein in multiple sclerosis and other neurological diseases: a comparative study. *Brain* 1999; 122 (Pt 11):2047-2056.
[95] Reindl M, Khalil M, Berger T. Antibodies as biological markers for pathophysiological processes in MS. *J Neuroimmunol* 2006; 180(1-2):50-62.
[96] Huizinga R, Linington C, Amor S. Resistance is futile: antineuronal autoimmunity in multiple sclerosis. *Trends Immunol* 2008; 29(2):54-60.
[97] Agius MA, Kirvan CA, Schafer AL, Gudipati E, Zhu S. High prevalence of anti-alpha-crystallin antibodies in multiple sclerosis: correlation with severity and activity of disease. *Acta Neurol Scand* 1999; 100(3):139-147.
[98] Williamson RA, Burgoon MP, Owens GP, Ghausi O, Leclerc E, Firme L, Carlson S, Corboy J, Parren PW, Sanna PP, Gilden DH, Burton DR. Anti-DNA antibodies are a major component of the intrathecal B cell response in multiple sclerosis. *Proc Natl Acad Sci* U S A 2001; 98(4):1793-1798.
[99] Tozzoli R. Recent advances in diagnostic technologies and their impact in autoimmune diseases. *Autoimmun Rev* 2007; 6(6):334-340.
[100] Plebani M, Pittoni M, Celadin M, Bernardi D, Mion MM. Recent advances in diagnostic technologies for autoimmune diseases. *Autoimmun Rev* 2009; 8(3):238-243.
[101] Blass S, Engel JM, Burmester GR. The immunologic homunculus in rheumatoid arthritis. *Arthritis Rheum* 1999; 42(12):2499-2506.
[102] Stinton LM, Fritzler MJ. A clinical approach to autoantibody testing in systemic autoimmune rheumatic disorders. *Autoimmun Rev* 2007; 7(1):77-84.
[103] Kanter JL, Narayana S, Ho PP, Catz I, Warren KG, Sobel RA, Steinman L, Robinson WH. Lipid microarrays identify key mediators of autoimmune brain inflammation. *Nat Med* 2006; 12(1):138-143.
[104] Quintana FJ, Farez MF, Viglietta V, Iglesias AH, Merbl Y, Izquierdo G, Lucas M, Basso AS, Khoury SJ, Lucchinetti CF, Cohen IR, Weiner HL. Antigen microarrays identify unique serum autoantibody signatures in clinical and pathologic subtypes of multiple sclerosis. *Proc Natl Acad Sci* U S A 2008; 105(48):18889-18894.
[105] Quintana FJ, Farez MF, Viglietta V, Iglesias AH, Merbl Y, Izquierdo G, Lucas M, Basso AS, Khoury SJ, Lucchinetti CF, Cohen IR, Weiner HL. Antigen microarrays identify unique serum autoantibody signatures in clinical and pathologic subtypes of multiple sclerosis. *Proc Natl Acad Sci* U S A 2008; 105(48):18889-18894.

[106] Cepok S, Zhou D, Srivastava R, Nessler S, Stei S, Bussow K, Sommer N, Hemmer B. Identification of Epstein-Barr virus proteins as putative targets of the immune response in multiple sclerosis. *J Clin Invest* 2005; 115(5):1352-1360.

[107] Cepok S, Zhou D, Srivastava R, Nessler S, Stei S, Bussow K, Sommer N, Hemmer B. Identification of Epstein-Barr virus proteins as putative targets of the immune response in multiple sclerosis. *J Clin Invest* 2005; 115(5):1352-1360.

[108] Lefranc D, Almeras L, Dubucquoi S, de Seze J, Vermersch P, Prin L. Distortion of the self-reactive IgG antibody repertoire in multiple sclerosis as a new diagnostic tool. *J Immunol* 2004; 172(1):669-678.

[109] Lefranc D, Almeras L, Dubucquoi S, de Seze J, Vermersch P, Prin L. Distortion of the self-reactive IgG antibody repertoire in multiple sclerosis as a new diagnostic tool. *J Immunol* 2004; 172(1):669-678.

[110] Kolln J, Ren HM, Da RR, Zhang Y, Spillner E, Olek M, Hermanowicz N, Hilgenberg LG, Smith MA, Van Den NS, Qin Y. Triosephosphate isomerase- and glyceraldehyde-3-phosphate dehydrogenase-reactive autoantibodies in the cerebrospinal fluid of patients with multiple sclerosis. *J Immunol* 2006; 177(8):5652-5658.

[111] Mathey EK, Derfuss T, Storch MK, Williams KR, Hales K, Woolley DR, Al Hayani A, Davies SN, Rasband MN, Olsson T, Moldenhauer A, Velhin S, Hohlfeld R, Meinl E, Linington C. Neurofascin as a novel target for autoantibody-mediated axonal injury. *J Exp Med* 2007; 204(10):2363-2372.

[112] Derfuss T, Parikh K, Velhin S, Braun M, Mathey E, Krumbholz M, Kumpfel T, Moldenhauer A, Rader C, Sonderegger P, Pollmann W, Tiefenthaller C, Bauer J, Lassmann H, Wekerle H, Karagogeos D, Hohlfeld R, Linington C, Meinl E. Contactin-2/TAG-1-directed autoimmunity is identified in multiple sclerosis patients and mediates gray matter pathology in animals. *Proc Natl Acad Sci* U S A 2009.

[113] Mathey EK, Derfuss T, Storch MK, Williams KR, Hales K, Woolley DR, Al Hayani A, Davies SN, Rasband MN, Olsson T, Moldenhauer A, Velhin S, Hohlfeld R, Meinl E, Linington C. Neurofascin as a novel target for autoantibody-mediated axonal injury. *J Exp Med* 2007; 204(10):2363-2372.

[114] Derfuss T, Parikh K, Velhin S, Braun M, Mathey E, Krumbholz M, Kumpfel T, Moldenhauer A, Rader C, Sonderegger P, Pollmann W, Tiefenthaller C, Bauer J, Lassmann H, Wekerle H, Karagogeos D, Hohlfeld R, Linington C, Meinl E. Contactin-2/TAG-1-directed autoimmunity is identified in multiple sclerosis patients and mediates gray matter pathology in animals. *Proc Natl Acad Sci* U S A 2009.

[115] Reindl M, Linington C, Brehm U, Egg R, Dilitz E, Deisenhammer F, Poewe W, Berger T. Antibodies against the myelin oligodendrocyte glycoprotein and the myelin basic protein in multiple sclerosis and other neurological diseases: a comparative study. *Brain* 1999; 122 (Pt 11):2047-2056.

[116] Olsson T, Baig S, Hojeberg B, Link H. Antimyelin basic protein and antimyelin antibody-producing cells in multiple sclerosis. *Ann Neurol* 1990; 27(2):132-136.

[117] Reindl M, Linington C, Brehm U, Egg R, Dilitz E, Deisenhammer F, Poewe W, Berger T. Antibodies against the myelin oligodendrocyte glycoprotein and the myelin basic protein in multiple sclerosis and other neurological diseases: a comparative study. *Brain* 1999; 122 (Pt 11):2047-2056.

[118] Moller JR, Johnson D, Brady RO, Tourtellotte WW, Quarles RH. Antibodies to myelin-associated glycoprotein (MAG) in the cerebrospinal fluid of multiple sclerosis patients. *J Neuroimmunol* 1989; 22(1):55-61.

[119] Sun JB, Olsson T, Wang WZ, Xiao BG, Kostulas V, Fredrikson S, Ekre HP, Link H. Autoreactive T and B cells responding to myelin proteolipid protein in multiple sclerosis and controls. *Eur J Immunol* 1991; 21(6):1461-1468.

[120] Lolli F, Mazzanti B, Pazzagli M, Peroni E, Alcaro MC, Sabatino G, Lanzillo R, Brescia M, V, Santoro L, Gasperini C, Galgani S, D'Elios MM, Zipoli V, Sotgiu S, Pugliatti M, Rovero P, Chelli M, Papini AM. The glycopeptide CSF114(Glc) detects serum antibodies in multiple sclerosis. *J Neuroimmunol* 2005; 167(1-2):131-137.

[121] Schwarz M, Spector L, Gortler M, Weisshaus O, Glass-Marmor L, Karni A, Dotan N, Miller A. Serum anti-Glc(alpha1,4)Glc(alpha) antibodies as a biomarker for relapsing-remitting multiple sclerosis. *J Neurol Sci* 2006; 244(1-2):59-68.

[122] Villar LM, Sadaba MC, Roldan E, Masjuan J, Gonzalez-Porque P, Villarrubia N, Espino M, Garcia-Trujillo JA, Bootello A, Alvarez-Cermeno JC. Intrathecal synthesis of oligoclonal IgM against myelin lipids predicts an aggressive disease course in MS. *J Clin Invest* 2005; 115(1):187-194.

[123] Kanter JL, Narayana S, Ho PP, Catz I, Warren KG, Sobel RA, Steinman L, Robinson WH. Lipid microarrays identify key mediators of autoimmune brain inflammation. *Nat Med* 2006; 12(1):138-143.

[124] Menge T, Lalive PH, von Budingen HC, Cree B, Hauser SL, Genain CP. Antibody responses against galactocerebroside are potential stage-specific biomarkers in multiple sclerosis. *J Allergy Clin Immunol* 2005; 116(2):453-459.

[125] Zanetta JP, Tranchant C, Kuchler-Bopp S, Lehmann S, Warter JM. Presence of anti-CSL antibodies in the cerebrospinal fluid of patients: a sensitive and specific test in the diagnosis of multiple sclerosis. *J Neuroimmunol* 1994; 52(2):175-182.

[126] Silber E, Semra YK, Gregson NA, Sharief MK. Patients with progressive multiple sclerosis have elevated antibodies to neurofilament subunit. *Neurology* 2002; 58(9):1372-1381.

[127] Sadatipour BT, Greer JM, Pender MP. Increased circulating antiganglioside antibodies in primary and secondary progressive multiple sclerosis. *Ann Neurol* 1998; 44(6):980-983.

[128] Rawes JA, Calabrese VP, Khan OA, DeVries GH. Antibodies to the axolemma-enriched fraction in the cerebrospinal fluid and serum of patients with multiple sclerosis and other neurological diseases. *Mult Scler* 1997; 3(6):363-369.

[129] Svarcova J, Fialova L, Bartos A, Steinbachova M, Malbohan I. Cerebrospinal fluid antibodies to tubulin are elevated in the patients with multiple sclerosis. *Eur J Neurol* 2008; 15(11):1173-1179.

[130] Reindl M, Khantane S, Ehling R, Schanda K, Lutterotti A, Brinkhoff C, Oertle T, Schwab ME, Deisenhammer F, Berger T, Bandtlow CE. Serum and cerebrospinal fluid antibodies to Nogo-A in patients with multiple sclerosis and acute neurological disorders. *J Neuroimmunol* 2003; 145(1-2):139-147.

[131] Onoue H, Satoh JI, Ogawa M, Tabunoki H, Yamamura T. Detection of anti-Nogo receptor autoantibody in the serum of multiple sclerosis and controls. *Acta Neurol Scand* 2007; 115(3):153-160.

[132] Lily O, Palace J, Vincent A. Serum autoantibodies to cell surface determinants in multiple sclerosis: a flow cytometric study. *Brain* 2004; 127(Pt 2):269-279.

[133] Mathey EK, Derfuss T, Storch MK, Williams KR, Hales K, Woolley DR, Al Hayani A, Davies SN, Rasband MN, Olsson T, Moldenhauer A, Velhin S, Hohlfeld R, Meinl E, Linington C. Neurofascin as a novel target for autoantibody-mediated axonal injury. *J Exp Med* 2007; 204(10):2363-2372.

[134] Derfuss T, Parikh K, Velhin S, Braun M, Mathey E, Krumbholz M, Kumpfel T, Moldenhauer A, Rader C, Sonderegger P, Pollmann W, Tiefenthaller C, Bauer J, Lassmann H, Wekerle H, Karagogeos D, Hohlfeld R, Linington C, Meinl E. Contactin-2/TAG-1-directed autoimmunity is identified in multiple sclerosis patients and mediates gray matter pathology in animals. *Proc Natl Acad Sci* U S A 2009.

[135] Lily O, Palace J, Vincent A. Serum autoantibodies to cell surface determinants in multiple sclerosis: a flow cytometric study. *Brain* 2004; 127(Pt 2):269-279.

[136] Niehaus A, Shi J, Grzenkowski M, Diers-Fenger M, Archelos J, Hartung HP, Toyka K, Bruck W, Trotter J. Patients with active relapsing-remitting multiple sclerosis synthesize antibodies recognizing oligodendrocyte progenitor cell surface protein: implications for remyelination. *Ann Neurol* 2000; 48(3):362-371.

[137] Bronstein JM, Lallone RL, Seitz RS, Ellison GW, Myers LW. A humoral response to oligodendrocyte-specific protein in MS: a potential molecular mimic. *Neurology* 1999; 53(1):154-161.

[138] Banki K, Colombo E, Sia F, Halladay D, Mattson DH, Tatum AH, Massa PT, Phillips PE, Perl A. Oligodendrocyte-specific expression and autoantigenicity of transaldolase in multiple sclerosis. *J Exp Med* 1994; 180(5):1649-1663.

[139] Walsh MJ, Murray JM. Dual implication of 2',3'-cyclic nucleotide 3' phosphodiesterase as major autoantigen and C3 complement-binding protein in the pathogenesis of multiple sclerosis. *J Clin Invest* 1998; 101(9):1923-1931.

[140] Agius MA, Kirvan CA, Schafer AL, Gudipati E, Zhu S. High prevalence of anti-alpha-crystallin antibodies in multiple sclerosis: correlation with severity and activity of disease. *Acta Neurol Scand* 1999; 100(3):139-147.

[141] Selmaj K, Brosnan CF, Raine CS. Expression of heat shock protein-65 by oligodendrocytes in vivo and in vitro: implications for multiple sclerosis. *Neurology* 1992; 42(4):795-800.

[142] Chiba S, Yokota S, Yonekura K, Tanaka S, Furuyama H, Kubota H, Fujii N, Matsumoto H. Autoantibodies against HSP70 family proteins were detected in the cerebrospinal fluid from patients with multiple sclerosis. *J Neurol Sci* 2006; 241(1-2):39-43.

[143] Cid C, Alvarez-Cermeno JC, Salinas M, Alcazar A. Anti-heat shock protein 90beta antibodies decrease pre-oligodendrocyte population in perinatal and adult cell cultures. Implications for remyelination in multiple sclerosis. *J Neurochem* 2005; 95(2):349-360.

[144] Mayo I, Arribas J, Villoslada P, Alvarez DR, Rodriguez-Vilarino S, Montalban X, De Sagarra MR, Castano JG. The proteasome is a major autoantigen in multiple sclerosis. *Brain* 2002; 125(Pt 12):2658-2667.

[145] Williamson RA, Burgoon MP, Owens GP, Ghausi O, Leclerc E, Firme L, Carlson S, Corboy J, Parren PW, Sanna PP, Gilden DH, Burton DR. Anti-DNA antibodies are a major component of the intrathecal B cell response in multiple sclerosis. *Proc Natl Acad Sci* USA 2001; 98(4):1793-1798.

[146] Sueoka E, Yukitake M, Iwanaga K, Sueoka N, Aihara T, Kuroda Y. Autoantibodies against heterogeneous nuclear ribonucleoprotein B1 in CSF of MS patients. *Ann Neurol* 2004; 56(6):778-786.

[147] Gorczyca WA, Ejma M, Witkowska D, Misiuk-Hojlo M, Kuropatwa M, Mulak M, Szymaniec S. Retinal antigens are recognized by antibodies present in sera of patients with multiple sclerosis. *Ophthalmic Res* 2004; 36(2):120-123.

[148] Kolln J, Ren HM, Da RR, Zhang Y, Spillner E, Olek M, Hermanowicz N, Hilgenberg LG, Smith MA, Van Den NS, Qin Y. Triosephosphate isomerase- and glyceraldehyde-3-phosphate dehydrogenase-reactive autoantibodies in the cerebrospinal fluid of patients with multiple sclerosis. *J Immunol* 2006; 177(8):5652-5658.

[149] Kolln J, Ren HM, Da RR, Zhang Y, Spillner E, Olek M, Hermanowicz N, Hilgenberg LG, Smith MA, Van Den NS, Qin Y. Triosephosphate isomerase- and glyceraldehyde-3-phosphate dehydrogenase-reactive autoantibodies in the cerebrospinal fluid of patients with multiple sclerosis. *J Immunol* 2006; 177(8):5652-5658.

[150] Archelos JJ, Trotter J, Previtali S, Weissbrich B, Toyka KV, Hartung HP. Isolation and characterization of an oligodendrocyte precursor-derived B-cell epitope in multiple sclerosis. *Ann Neurol* 1998; 43(1):15-24.

[151] Cepok S, Zhou D, Srivastava R, Nessler S, Stei S, Bussow K, Sommer N, Hemmer B. Identification of Epstein-Barr virus proteins as putative targets of the immune response in multiple sclerosis. *J Clin Invest* 2005; 115(5):1352-1360.

[152] Cepok S, Zhou D, Srivastava R, Nessler S, Stei S, Bussow K, Sommer N, Hemmer B. Identification of Epstein-Barr virus proteins as putative targets of the immune response in multiple sclerosis. *J Clin Invest* 2005; 115(5):1352-1360.

[153] Reindl M, Khalil M, Berger T. Antibodies as biological markers for pathophysiological processes in MS. *J Neuroimmunol* 2006; 180(1-2):50-62.

[154] Huizinga R, Linington C, Amor S. Resistance is futile: antineuronal autoimmunity in multiple sclerosis. *Trends Immunol* 2008; 29(2):54-60.

[155] Archelos JJ, Trotter J, Previtali S, Weissbrich B, Toyka KV, Hartung HP. Isolation and characterization of an oligodendrocyte precursor-derived B-cell epitope in multiple sclerosis. *Ann Neurol* 1998; 43(1):15-24.

[156] Archelos JJ, Trotter J, Previtali S, Weissbrich B, Toyka KV, Hartung HP. Isolation and characterization of an oligodendrocyte precursor-derived B-cell epitope in multiple sclerosis. *Ann Neurol* 1998; 43(1):15-24.

[157] Owens GP, Burgoon MP, Devlin ME, Gilden DH. Strategies to identify sequences or antigens unique to multiple sclerosis. *Mult Scler* 1996; 2(4):184-194.

[158] Smith GP. Filamentous fusion phage: novel expression vectors that display cloned antigens on the virion surface. *Science* 1985; 228(4705):1315-1317.

[159] Smith GP. Filamentous fusion phage: novel expression vectors that display cloned antigens on the virion surface. *Science* 1985; 228(4705):1315-1317.

[160] Webster R. Biology of the Filamentous Bacteriophage. In: Kay B, Winter J, McCafferty J, editors. *Phage Display of Peptides and Proteins. A laboratory Manual.* San Diego, California: Academic Press, INC, 1996: 1-20.

[161] Smith GP. Filamentous fusion phage: novel expression vectors that display cloned antigens on the virion surface. *Science* 1985; 228(4705):1315-1317.

[162] Archelos JJ, Trotter J, Previtali S, Weissbrich B, Toyka KV, Hartung HP. Isolation and characterization of an oligodendrocyte precursor-derived B-cell epitope in multiple sclerosis. *Ann Neurol* 1998; 43(1):15-24.

[163] Owens GP, Burgoon MP, Devlin ME, Gilden DH. Strategies to identify sequences or antigens unique to multiple sclerosis. *Mult Scler* 1996; 2(4):184-194.

[164] Scott JK, Smith GP. Searching for peptide ligands with an epitope library. *Science* 1990; 249(4967):386-390.

[165] Cortese I, Tafi R, Grimaldi LM, Martino G, Nicosia A, Cortese R. Identification of peptides specific for cerebrospinal fluid antibodies in multiple sclerosis by using phage libraries. *Proc Natl Acad Sci* U S A 1996; 93(20):11063-11067.

[166] Cortese I, Capone S, Luchetti S, Grimaldi LM, Nicosia A, Cortese R. CSF-enriched antibodies do not share specificities among MS patients. *Mult Scler* 1998; 4(3):118-123.

[167] Dybwad A, Flrre O, Sioud M. Probing for cerebrospinal fluid antibody specificities by a panel of random peptide libraries. *Autoimmunity* 1997; 25(2):85-89.

[168] Jolivet-Reynaud C, Perron H, Ferrante P, Becquart L, Dalbon P, Mandrand B. Specificities of multiple sclerosis cerebrospinal fluid and serum antibodies against mimotopes. *Clin Immunol* 1999; 93(3):283-293.

[169] Rand KH, Houck H, Denslow ND, Heilman KM. Molecular approach to find target(s) for oligoclonal bands in multiple sclerosis. *J Neurol Neurosurg Psychiatry* 1998; 65(1):48-55.

[170] Rand KH, Houck H, Denslow ND, Heilman KM. Epstein-Barr virus nuclear antigen-1 (EBNA-1) associated oligoclonal bands in patients with multiple sclerosis. *J Neurol Sci* 2000; 173(1):32-39.

[171] Cortese I, Capone S, Luchetti S, Cortese R, Nicosia A. Cross-reactive phage-displayed mimotopes lead to the discovery of mimicry between HSV-1 and a brain-specific protein. *J Neuroimmunol* 2001; 113(1):119-128.

[172] Cortese I, Capone S, Luchetti S, Cortese R, Nicosia A. Cross-reactive phage-displayed mimotopes lead to the discovery of mimicry between HSV-1 and a brain-specific protein. *J Neuroimmunol* 2001; 113(1):119-128.

[173] Hufton SE, Moerkerk PT, Meulemans EV, de Bruine A, Arends JW, Hoogenboom HR. Phage display of cDNA repertoires: the pVI display system and its applications for the selection of immunogenic ligands. *J Immunol Methods* 1999; 231(1-2):39-51.

[174] Becker KG, Mattson DH, Powers JM, Gado AM, Biddison WE. Analysis of a sequenced cDNA library from multiple sclerosis lesions. *J Neuroimmunol* 1997; 77(1):27-38.

[175] Becker KG, Mattson DH, Powers JM, Gado AM, Biddison WE. Analysis of a sequenced cDNA library from multiple sclerosis lesions. *J Neuroimmunol* 1997; 77(1):27-38.

[176] Becker KG, Mattson DH, Powers JM, Gado AM, Biddison WE. Analysis of a sequenced cDNA library from multiple sclerosis lesions. *J Neuroimmunol* 1997; 77(1):27-38.

[177] Somers V, Govarts C, Somers K, Hupperts R, Medaer R, Stinissen P. Autoantibody profiling in multiple sclerosis reveals novel antigenic candidates. *J Immunol* 2008; 180(6):3957-3963.

[178] Somers V, Govarts C, Somers K, Hupperts R, Medaer R, Stinissen P. Autoantibody profiling in multiple sclerosis reveals novel antigenic candidates. *J Immunol* 2008; 180(6):3957-3963.
[179] Link H, Baig S, Jiang YP, Olsson O, Hojeberg B, Kostulas V, Olsson T. B cells and antibodies in MS. *Res Immunol* 1989; 140(2):219-226.
[180] Sun J, Link H, Olsson T, Xiao BG, Andersson G, Ekre HP, Linington C, Diener P. T and B cell responses to myelin-oligodendrocyte glycoprotein in multiple sclerosis. *J Immunol* 1991; 146(5):1490-1495.
[181] Lambracht-Washington D, O'connor KC, Cameron EM, Jowdry A, Ward ES, Frohman E, Racke MK, Monson NL. Antigen specificity of clonally expanded and receptor edited cerebrospinal fluid B cells from patients with relapsing remitting MS. *J Neuroimmunol* 2007.
[182] von Budingen HC, Harrer MD, Kuenzle S, Meier M, Goebels N. Clonally expanded plasma cells in the cerebrospinal fluid of MS patients produce myelin-specific antibodies. *Eur J Immunol* 2008; 38(7):2014-2023.
[183] Zhang Y, Da RR, Guo W, Ren HM, Hilgenberg LG, Sobel RA, Tourtellotte WW, Smith MA, Olek M, Gupta S, Robertson RT, Nagra R, van den NS, Qin Y. Axon reactive B cells clonally expanded in the cerebrospinal fluid of patients with multiple sclerosis. *J Clin Immunol* 2005; 25(3):254-264.
[184] Kolln J, Ren HM, Da RR, Zhang Y, Spillner E, Olek M, Hermanowicz N, Hilgenberg LG, Smith MA, van den NS, Qin Y. Triosephosphate isomerase- and glyceraldehyde-3-phosphate dehydrogenase-reactive autoantibodies in the cerebrospinal fluid of patients with multiple sclerosis. *J Immunol* 2006; 177(8):5652-5658.
[185] Yu X, Gilden D, Schambers L, Barmina O, Burgoon M, Bennett J, Owens G. Peptide reactivity between multiple sclerosis (MS) CSF IgG and recombinant antibodies generated from clonally expanded plasma cells in MS CSF. *J Neuroimmunol* 2010.
[186] Martin DR, Marlowe RL, Ahearn JM. Determination of the role for CD21 during Epstein-Barr virus infection of B-lymphoblastoid cells. *J Virol* 1994; 68(8):4716-4726.
[187] Sugimoto M, Tahara H, Ide T, Furuichi Y. Steps involved in immortalization and tumorigenesis in human B-lymphoblastoid cell lines transformed by Epstein-Barr virus. *Cancer Res* 2004; 64(10):3361-3364.
[188] Roughan JE, Torgbor C, Thorley-Lawson DA. Germinal center B cells latently infected with Epstein-Barr virus proliferate extensively but do not increase in number. *J Virol* 2010; 84(2):1158-1168.
[189] Counter CM, Botelho FM, Wang P, Harley CB, Bacchetti S. Stabilization of short telomeres and telomerase activity accompany immortalization of Epstein-Barr virus-transformed human B lymphocytes. *J Virol* 1994; 68(5):3410-3414.
[190] Satoh M, Yasuda T, Higaki T, Goto M, Tanuma S, Ide T, Furuichi Y, Sugimoto M. Innate apoptosis of human B lymphoblasts transformed by Epstein-Barr virus: modulation by cellular immortalization and senescence. *Cell Struct Funct* 2003; 28(1):61-70.
[191] Morin GB. The human telomere terminal transferase enzyme is a ribonucleoprotein that synthesizes TTAGGG repeats. *Cell* 1989; 59(3):521-529.
[192] Sugimoto M, Ide T, Goto M, Furuichi Y. Reconsideration of senescence, immortalization and telomere maintenance of Epstein-Barr virus-transformed human B-lymphoblastoid cell lines. *Mech Ageing Dev* 1999; 107(1):51-60.

[193] Sugimoto M, Furuichi Y, Ide T, Goto M. Incorrect us of "immortalization" for B-lymphoblastoid cell lines transformed by Epstein-Barr virus. *J Virol* 1999; 73(11):9690-9691.

[194] Takahashi T, Kawabe T, Okazaki Y, Itoh C, Noda K, Tajima M, Satoh M, Goto M, Mitsui Y, Tahara H, Ide T, Furuichi Y, Sugimoto M. In vitro establishment of tumorigenic human B-lymphoblastoid cell lines transformed by Epstein-Barr virus. *DNA Cell Biol* 2003; 22(11):727-735.

[195] Shiratori M, Sakamoto S, Suzuki N, Tokutake Y, Kawabe Y, Enomoto T, Sugimoto M, Goto M, Matsumoto T, Furuichi Y. Detection by epitope-defined monoclonal antibodies of Werner DNA helicases in the nucleoplasm and their upregulation by cell transformation and immortalization. *J Cell Biol* 1999; 144(1):1-9.

[196] Okada M, Goto M, Furuichi Y, Sugimoto M. Differential effects of cytotoxic drugs on mortal and immortalized B-lymphoblastoid cell lines from normal and Werner's syndrome patients. *Biol Pharm Bull* 1998; 21(3):235-239.

[197] Fraussen J, Vrolix K, Martinez-Martinez P, Losen M, Meulemans E, De Baets MH, Stinissen P, Somers V. A novel method for making human monoclonal antibodies. *J Autoimmun* 2010; 35(2):130-134.

[198] Fraussen J, Vrolix K, Martinez-Martinez P, Hupperts R, Van Diepen A, Meulemans E, De Baets M, Stinissen P, Somers V. Antibody-producing Monoclonal B Cell Lines from Multiple Sclerosis Patients Obtained by B Cell Immortalization. *Clinical Immunology* 2009; 131:S129-S130.

[199] Fraussen J, Martinez P, De Baets M, Van Diepen A, Meulemans E, Stinissen P, Somers V. Characterizing autoantibodies in multiple sclerosis by B cell immortalization. *Journal of Neuroimmunology* 2008; 203(2):183-184.

[200] Vrolix K, Fraussen J, Meulemans E, Becker P, Phernambucq M, Somers V, Losen M, De Baets M, Martinez Martinez P. Monoclonal antibody production by immortalization of B cells from the thymus of myasthenia gravis patients. *Journal of Neuroimmunology* 2008; 203(2):258.

In: Multiple Sclerosis
Editor: E. Scholz and C. Müller, pp. 31-57

ISBN 978-1-61324-848-5

Chapter II

Multiple Sclerosis: The Role of Fatty Acids

***Gloudina M. Hon*[1] *and Tandi Matsha*[1,*]**
[1]Department of Bio-Medical Sciences, Faculty of Health and Wellness Science, Cape Peninsula University of Technology, P O Box 1906, Bellville, 7530, Cape Town, South Africa

Abstract

Multiple sclerosis is a chronic inflammatory disease of the central nervous system which leads to neuronal demyelination. As the disease progresses, oligodendrocytes and axons are destroyed, resulting in sclerotic plaques, or lesion formation. Although treatment is available that can alleviate some of the symptoms, no cure is available. Therefore, as more lesions are formed in the brain, nerve impulse transmission becomes progressively impaired, and brain functions are increasingly compromised, resulting in a gradual decline in health and quality of life. The underlying cause of multiple sclerosis remains unknown, but both an autoimmune and an infectious aetiology are suspected, both of which would initiate the inflammatory process. Genetic factors may also contribute to the disease aetiology. Metabolic disturbances, especially lipid metabolic abnormalities, have also been implicated in the aetiology of the disease. Although the reports are inconsistent, particularly C18:2n-6 (linoleic acid) and C20:4n-6 (arachidonic acid) have been shown to be reduced in the plasma, platelets, white and red blood cells, and CSF from patients with multiple sclerosis. These fatty acids are precursors for pro-inflammatory eicosanoid production, which are reported to be increased during the inflammatory response in neurodegenerative diseases. Eicosanoids regulate cellular functions, but their effects also depend on each precursor fatty acid and the cell type concerned. Inflammation is a defence mechanism of the body against various insults,

* Corresponding author: Tandi Matsha (PhD), Biomedical Technology, Faculty of Health and Wellness Science, Cape Peninsula University of Technology, P O Box 1906, Bellville, 7535 Cape Town, South Africa. Telephone number: + 27 21 959 6366; Fax number: +27 21 959 6760; E-mail address: matshat@cput.ac.za.

which is usually a well-controlled process, although it may be accompanied by some damage to surrounding tissue.

1.1. Introduction

Multiple sclerosis (MS) is a chronic inflammatory disease of the central nervous system (CNS) which leads to neuronal demyelination. As the disease progresses, oligodendrocytes and axons are destroyed, resulting in sclerotic plaques, or lesion formation (Brück, 2005; Adibhatla & Hatcher, 2007). The underlying cause of MS remains unknown, but both an autoimmune and an infectious aetiology are suspected. Genetic factors may also contribute to the disease etiology (Cooper, 1997; Stinissen et al. 1997; Hunter & Hafler, 2000; Brown, 2001; Chatzimanolis et al. 2004; Brück, 2005; Adibhatla & Hatcher, 2007). Metabolic disturbances, especially lipid metabolic abnormalities, have also been implicated in the development of the disease (Baker et al. 1964; Cumings et al. 1965; Cunnane et al. 1989; Lassmann et al. 2001; Harbige & Sharief, 2007). Although treatment is available that can alleviate some of the symptoms, no cure is available. Therefore, as more lesions are formed in the brain, nerve impulse transmission becomes progressively impaired, and brain functions are increasingly compromised. As the disease develops, patients with MS experience a gradual decline in health and quality of life (Jelinek, 2000; Brown, 2001; Brück, 2005).

1.2. Epidemiology of Multiple Sclerosis

Multiple sclerosis is a relatively newly recognised disease. A few cases of MS were reported in the beginning of the 19th century, but the disease was recognised as a clinical disease only as late as 1860 (Compston & Coles, 2002). Currently, the disease is one of the more common neurological diseases. Worldwide, an estimated 2.5 million people have MS and the disease has an incidence and prevalence of 7 per 100,000 and 120 per 100,000 respectively, with a lifetime risk of 1 in 400 (Jelinek, 2000; Compston & Coles, 2002). There is a wide geographic variation in the prevalence of MS, with the highest in Northern Europe, Southern Australia, the middle part of North America and the United Kingdom (Jelinek, 2000; Noseworthy et al. 2000; Reipert, 2004). In the United Kingdom the incidence of MS is approximately 1 in 800 people and in northern Europe 1 in 1000. There is scarcity of literature on the prevalence and incidence of MS in the developing countries, including South Africa (Modi et al. 2008). However, a recent study on 430 patients with MS living in South Africa and based on patient-orientated questionnaires, presented similar findings to those reported in the literature (Modi et al. 2008).

According to recent studies, MS is the most common disease of the CNS of inflammatory and demyelinating origin, and also the most common neurological disorder in young adults (Jelinek, 2000; Compston & Coles, 2002; Reipert, 2004; Leary et al. 2005; Okuda et al. 2005). Its onset is usually between 20 and 40 years of age, but about 5 % of patients are diagnosed before the age of 16 years. Females are more susceptible than males, with a ratio of about 2 to 1. Susceptibility to MS varies between different racial and ethnic groups. The disease is rare among North and South Amerindians, Chinese, Japanese, African blacks and

New Zealand Maoris (Rosati, 2001). This difference in susceptibility to MS has resulted in an uneven geographic distribution of the disease. However, prevalence studies also show lower prevalence of MS among white people outside Europe than in many parts of northern Europe (Compston & Coles, 2002), and increased susceptibility in first-generation black people in the United Kingdom. One of the possible explanations for the differences in these surveys are said to be due to improved case recognition in the developed countries. This cannot explain the phenomenon for example that English-speaking people who migrate to South Africa as adults have a higher risk of developing MS than those who migrate as children (Compston & Coles, 2002). These findings suggested that an environmental factor could be contributing to the development of the disease.

1.3. Types of Multiple Sclerosis

There are a number of internationally recognized forms of MS, such as relapsing remitting multiple sclerosis (RRMS), secondary progressive multiple sclerosis (SPMS) and primary progressive multiple sclerosis (PPMS). About 80% of people presenting with MS are diagnosed with RRMS. About 50% of these patients will progress to SPMS within 10 years of disease onset. This figure increases to about 90% over the next 25 to 30 years. Another 10 to 20 % of people presenting with MS are diagnosed with PPMS (Lublin & Reingold, 1996; Reipert, 2004). Patients with RRMS experience a series of relapses, each followed by a complete or partial remission of symptoms. The duration and frequency of relapses vary, and recovery can be gradual or fast (Lublin & Reingold, 1996; Reipert, 2004). Secondary progressive multiple sclerosis (SPMS) is characterized by a steady progression of neurological deterioration. Patients may experience relapses, minor remissions and plateaus, but these may also be absent (Lublin & Reingold, 1996; Reipert, 2004). Primary progressive multiple sclerosis (PPMS) is characterized by a gradual progression of the disease that leads to a decline in the patients physical abilities. These patients experience only short periods of minor remissions of symptoms (Lublin & Reingold, 1996; Reipert, 2004).

1.4. Symptoms

Patients with MS can experience loss of any function that is controlled by the CNS. Clinical features include loss of sensation, muscle weakness, spasticity, visual loss, in-coordination, cognitive impairment, pain, as well as bladder and bowel disturbances (Noseworthy et al. 2000; Chwastiak et al. 2002; Compston & Coles, 2002; Reipert, 2004; Leary et al. 2005). Many patients also experience fatigue, which is accompanied by increases in body temperature. Patients with MS also take longer to recover from both physical and cognitive tasks. In time, symptoms such as cognitive impairment, vertigo, spasticity, ataxia tremors, progressive quadriparesis, pain and depression may become excessive. As patients become more disabled, their quality of life deteriorates and they may become an economic burden on society (Adibhatla & Hatcher, 2007). Life expectancy of MS patients is at least 25 years from disease onset, and many patients die from unrelated causes (Compston & Coles, 2002).

1.5. Diagnosis

Diagnostic criteria for MS (McDonald Diagnostic Criteria) were updated in 2001 and revised in 2005. These criteria include the integration of magnetic resonance image assessment (MRI) with clinical and para-clinical methods (Reipert, 2004; Polman et al. 2005). The 2005 revised diagnostic criteria for MS specify that at least two neurological events must occur before diagnosis may be established. These events or relapses must be separated in time and also anatomically. The presence of multifocal lesions of various ages are evaluated together with additional tests such as cerebrospinal fluid (CSF) analysis and visual evoked potential (VEP) recordings, before a final diagnosis can be made (Noseworthy et al. 2000; Chwastiak et al. 2002; Reipert, 2004; Polman et al. 2005). Once diagnosis of MS is confirmed, the degree of disability can be monitored, using the Kurtzke Expanded Disability Status Scale (EDSS) (Kurtzke, 1983; Reipert, 2004).

1.5.1. Kurtzke Expanded Disability Status Scale

The functional disability status (disease severity) of patients with MS can be measured using the Kurtzke Expanded Disability Status Scale (EDSS), which includes eight Functional Systems (FS). The Functional Systems are Pyramidal, Cerebellar, Brainstem, Sensory, Bowel and bladder, Visual, Cerebral and "other" (Kurtzke, 1983; Reipert, 2004). The EDSS, as well as the Functional Systems, are assigned a Functional System Score (FSS) by investigating neurologists. Higher values indicate greater disability. Scales for the EDSS are from 0 to 10, in which the 0 score indicates no disability at all and 10 indicates death due to MS.

1.6. Treatment

Neurodegenerative diseases, including MS, are of clinical importance because neurons regenerate slowly (Brown, 2001; Pino et al. 2005; Adibhatla & Hatcher, 2007). Neuronal remyelination in MS is limited, resulting in the multifocal sclerotic plaques from which the disease gets its name (Compston & Coles, 2002). Currently, there are treatments available to slow the course of the disease and alleviate the symptoms, but none that could cure the disease. Treatment of MS is mostly based on alleviation of inflammation, but the effects of these on the immune system have not been fully investigated (Compston & Coles, 2002; Reipert, 2004; Van Meeteren et al. 2005; Schippling et al. 2008).

Drugs that are able to modify the course of the disease (disease-modifiers) that have been approved for the treatment of MS are interferon beta, glatiramer acetate, mitoxantrone and corticosteroids (Compston & Coles, 2002; Reipert, 2004). Interferon-β and glatiramer acetate are both immuno-modulatory drugs, while mitoxantrone and cyclophosphamide are immunosuppressive drugs (Schippling et al. 2008) Interferon-β1b has been approved in the treatment of RRMS as it decreases the clinical relapse rate and disease activity and severity (Chatzimanolis et al. 2004). Corticosteroids are anti-inflammatory and have been used for acute treatment of MS relapses (Compston & Coles, 2002). However, the efficiency of these drugs in suppressing inflammation and clinical relapses in patients with MS is limited (Schippling et al. 2008).

Recent studies have shown promising results on the use of haemopoietic stem-cell transplantation in the treatment of severe forms of MS (Fassas et al. 2000; Fassas et al. 2002; Schippling et al. 2008), but the effectiveness of this treatment still needs to be evaluated in large randomized, prospective controlled trials. Although the mortality rate has dropped to about 1-2 % of treated cases, stem-cell transplantation therapy is still considered to be potentially a life-threatening procedure (Mancardi & Saccardi, 2008; Schippling et al. 2008).

Various membrane fatty acid metabolic abnormalities have been reported in patients with MS, especially fatty acids known to be involved in the inflammatory process, such as the n-6 (omega-6) and n-3 (omega-3) polyunsaturated fatty acids (PUFAs) (Cumings et al. 1965; Cherayil, 1984; Fisher et al. 1987; Navarro & Segura, 1989; Harbige & Sharief, 2007). Subsequently, a number of studies have evaluated the use of fatty acid supplementation in the treatment of MS. In general, improvement in neurological outcome in these patients was measured against a reduction in the EDSS, as well as against exacerbation rate and duration. Several studies reported an improvement in symptoms during n-6 and n-3 fatty acid supplementation (Bates et al. 1978; Nordvik et al. 2000; Weinstock-Guttman et al. 2005; Harbige & Sharief, 2007). There were also reports with negative results (Paty et al. 1978) and a recent Cochrane review of all randomized trials of dietary regimens for MS, showed that PUFAs did not have a significant effect on disease progression as measured by the Disability Status Scale (Farinotti et al. 2007). The risk of developing MS is also associated with increased dietary intake of saturated fatty acids (Van Meeteren et al. 2005), but similar to findings for PUFA supplementation in MS, results from a prospective study showed that the amount and type of dietary fat, including saturated fatty acids, showed no affect on the risk of developing MS (Westlund & Kurland, 1953; Antonovsky et al. 1965; Cendrowski et al. 1969; Warren et al. 1982; Butcher, 1986; Zhang et al. 2000).

1.7. The Aetiology of Multiple Sclerosis

The inflammatory response can be initiated by different factors, such as microbiological, immunological and toxic agents (Simopoulos, 2002). Findings on the mechanisms involved in MS development are inconclusive, but include the possibility of an autoimmune response, virus mediation, and metabolic disturbances. Some findings seem to suggest that metabolic disturbances could be responsible for primary oligodendrocyte damage, preceding auto-immune responses (Martino & Hartung, 1999; Lassmann et al. 2001; Hafler, 2004; Matute & Perez-Cerda, 2005; Harbige & Sharief, 2007). In MS, oligodendrocytes, the cells which synthesize and maintain the protective myelin sheath around neuronal axons, are the principal target of immune attack (Compston & Coles, 2002), whereas microglial cells, B and T lymphocytes, and macrophages are involved in the inflammatory response (Prineas & Wright, 1978; Bjartmar & Trapp, 2001; Brown, 2001; Brück, 2005; Adibhatla & Hatcher, 2007).

1.7.1. Inflammation

Inflammation is a defense mechanism of the body against various insults, which is usually a well-controlled process, although it may be accompanied by some damage to surrounding tissue (Brown, 2001; Calder, 2001; Kulmatycki & Jamali, 2006; Farooqui et al. 2007). The initial inflammatory response, innate immunity, is non-specific, and does not need previous exposure to pathogens to be activated (Rola-Pleszezynski & Stankova, 1992; Calder, 2001). Innate immunity functions by the elimination of pathogens by compliment, toxic chemicals released by phagocytes, toxic proteins released by natural killer cells, or phagocytosis by macrophages (Calder, 2001). Acquired immunity, in contrast to innate immunity, involves the recognition of antigens on invading pathogens. Lymphocytes form a part of the acquired immune response; humoral immunity involves B-lymphocytes, which deal with extra-cellular pathogens through antibody production, while T-lymphocytes are part of a cell-mediated system, in which intra-cellular pathogens are dealt with. T-lymphocytes function by recognizing antigens, together with major histocompatibility complex (MHC) molecules, displayed on cell surfaces of antigen presenting cells, such as macrophages, dendritic cells and B-lymphocytes (Calder, 2001). Re-infection by the same pathogen will result in a stronger and faster response.

Communication within the immune system is through direct cell-to-cell contact, involving adhesion molecules, and by the production of two classes of chemical messengers, cytokines and eicosanoids. Cytokines are synthesized by phagocytes and parenchymal cells. These messengers can alter the activity of target cells by binding to specific receptors on the cell surface of these cells. Eicosanoids are derived from cell membrane PUFAs, and modulate the more specific acquired immune response (Horrobin & Manku, 1990; Rola-Pleszezynski & Stankova, 1992; Calder, 2001; Bagga et al. 2003; Zamaria, 2004). To this group belong prostaglandins (PGs), leukotrienes (LTs), thromboxanes (TXs) and platelet activating factor (PAF). They are produced soon after stimulation and regulate many inflammatory effects, such as induction of fever, vasodilation, and production of macrophage- and lymphocyte-derived cytokines. They also modulate immune cell functions (De Pablo & De Cienfuegos, 2000; Tilley et al. 2001).

Glial cells are distributed throughout the CNS and are important cells for the survival of existing neurons. These cells include oligodendrocytes, microglia and astrocytes (Matute et al. 2001; Miller, 2005; Farooqui et al. 2007). Microglia are the main mediators of neuro-inflammation and are responsible for the recruitment of leukocytes from the blood stream into brain tissue. When activated, they migrate to injured sites where they remove dead cells through phagocytosis. Inflammatory responses usually result in self-limiting healing processes. In patients with MS, however, this leads to apoptosis of oligodendrocytes and lesion formation, causing the relapses experienced by patients. In this regard, glial involvement has been shown in CNS disorders, especially in MS. Barnett and Prineas (2004) reported that during the first few hours of the formation of a new lesion, microglia were the only immune cells present in the apoptotic zone, while T-lymphocytes, early activated macrophages and myelin phagocytes were rare or absent in the apoptotic zone, although they were present elsewhere in the lesion (Gay et al. 1997; Aboul-Enein, et al. 2003; Barnett & Prineas, 2004). Prineas and Wright (1978) have reported plasma cells (differentiated B-lymphocytes) to be present as well; both in MS normal white matter, but with increased numbers in chronic plague tissue.

1.7.1.1. Markers of Inflammation

There are several recognised markers of inflammation which include serum soluble vascular adhesion molecule-1 (sVCAM-1), soluble intercellular adhesion molecule-1 (sICAM-1), C-reactive protein (CRP), neopterin, serum nitric oxide metabolites nitrate and nitrite, tumour necrosis factor alpha (TNF-α) and alpha 1-acid glycoprotein (AGP) (Giovannoni et al. 2001; Adam et al. 2003; Henry et al. 2003; Weinstock-Guttman et al. 2005). Of these CRP is a marker of choice because its assay is commonly available in the routine biochemistry laboratories. CRP as an acute phase protein is wildely used as a marker of both infection and inflammation. It has also been used as a pro-inflammatory marker in assessment of the degree of inflammation in patients with MS (Giovannoni et al. 2001; Sellner et al. 2008). A disadvantage of using serum inflammatory markers is that they don't always correlate with short-term disease progression (Giovannoni et al. 2001), but they have been shown to correlate with infectious episodes and clinical relapse in MS patients (Giovannoni et al. 1996).

1.7.2. Infectious Agents in Multiple Sclerosis

More than 20 infectious agents have been reported to be associated with MS; but these associations have never been confirmed to be a direct cause of the disease. However, exposure to infectious agents in early childhood has been reported as a contributing factor which could initiate the onset of MS. Furthermore, relapses in MS frequently follow gastrointestinal or upper respiratory tract infections (Karpuj et al. 1997). There are different theories explaining virus action in the chronic inflammatory condition of patients with MS. One possibility is that certain microbes can mimic myelin fragments and can therefore trigger the immune response. Another theory involves superantigens, which are toxins produced by certain viruses and which can directly interact with T-lymphocyte receptors to trigger an inflammatory reaction (Karpuj et al. 1997; Willer & Ebers, 2000; Moses & Sriram, 2001).

Viruses that have been implicated in susceptibility to MS include both endogenous and exogenous viruses and range from retroviruses to herpes viruses and measles. Multiple sclerosis-associated retrovirus/human endogenous retrovirus W (MSRV/HERV-W) and Human herpesvirus-6 (HHV-6) are the two most studied viruses as environmental co-factors in MS (Mameli et al. 2007). Other exogenous viruses such as Epstein-Barr virus (EBV), Varicella Zoster virus (VZV) and JC virus (JCV) have been implicated in the disease as well. Results are varied, but in general higher virus presence and expression in MS than in healthy subjects have been reported.

1.7.2.1. Exogenous Viruses

Mancuso et al. (2007) found that HHV-6 and JCV were present in the CSF of patients with MS and other neurological diseases (OND), whereas Mameli et al. (2007) reported no difference between patients with MS and healthy controls with regards to presence and replication of HHV-6 in the brain or peripheral blood mononuclear cells. Mancuso et al. (2007) reported the presence of VZV in the CSF of a subgroup of patients with MS, but absent in the CSF of normal controls and that of other neurological disorders. The absence of VZV in some of the patients with MS showed the lack of a causative effect of VZV in the aetiology of MS however. Infectious mononucleosis (caused by EBV infection) has also been implicated as a risk factor in MS development, and furthermore this risk may persist for at least 30 years after the initial infection (Nielsen et al. 2007).

1.7.2.2. Endogenous Viruses

Inherited retroviruses such as MSRV/HERV-W are present in the human brain in healthy subjects, but in patients with MS they are actively expressed (Perron et al. 2005; Sotgiu et al. 2006; Mameli et al. 2007). Converging results from three independent groups, Perron et al. (2005) showed this difference in MSRV/HERV-W GAG and ENV antigen expression (proteins) between normal and MS brains. These differences could be a reflection of differential regulation of inherited HERV-W copies, or expression of "infectious" MSRV copies. The presence of MSRV virions in the CSF from patients with early onset MS, was associated with a worse prognosis in follow-up studies (Sotgiu et al. 2006). De Villiers et al. (2006) reported expression of MSRV pol gene in the serum of 69 % of patients with MS, but also in 70 % of unaffected close relatives of the patients.

Reports indicate that the endogenous virus HERV-W is active in patients with MS. Antony et al. (2004) reported that syncytin was expressed in microglia and astrocytes from patients with MS. Syncytin is a virus-expressed glycoprotein that can induce the release of redox reactants, which are cytotoxic to cells (Antony et al. 2004). Astrocytes, which recycle the neurotransmitter glutamate (Piani & Fontana, 1994; Miller, 2005; Van Meeteren et al. 2005), abandon this function when they are injured. Increased concentrations of glutamate cause over-activation of glutamate receptors on oligodendrocytes, which may result in cell death (Oka et al. 1993; Matute et al. 2001; Van Meeteren et al. 2005).

1.7.3. Genetic Factors

Autoimmune diseases may be the result of an interaction between environmental factors and multiple, specific genes (Karpuj et al. 1997; Willer & Ebers, 2000). The development of MS may also be associated with genetic factors, as was shown by an increased relative risk of this disease in siblings when compared to the general population. Several regions of the human genome are associated with susceptibility to MS, but the impact of environmental conditions still needs clarification (Karpuj et al. 1997). The identification of genes that impart susceptibility to a disease is of great importance as this may result in finding preventive measures and improved therapy (Karpuj et al. 1997).

The genetic analysis of MS has been based mainly on studies in which the sharing of certain alleles of candidate genes in unrelated affected individuals is compared with that of a control population (Karpuj et al. 1997; Noseworthy et al. 2000; Willer & Ebers, 2000). Since MS is an inflammatory disease, the focus has therefore been on genes which are involved in the immune response. Zeis et al. (2007) reported that in brain tissue from patients with MS, consistent up-regulation of genes involved with anti-inflammatory and protective mechanisms, such as signal transducer and activator of transcription 6 (STAT6), Janus kinases (JAKI), interleukin 4 receptor (IL-4R), Interleukin 10 (IL-10), Chromogranin C and hypoxia-inducible factor (Hif-Iα), were expressed mainly by oligodendrocytes. In contrast, genes involved in pro-inflammatory mechanisms, such as STAT4, interleukin Iβ (IL-Iβ) and macrophage colony-stimulating factor (MCSF) were predominantly up-regulated in microglia (Zeis et al. 2007). Up-regulation of genes involved in anti-inflammatory mechanisms may protect the CNS environment, whereas the activation of pro-inflammatory mechanisms in microglia may favour disease progression. Other immune responsive genes include the major histocompatibility complex (MHC) on chromosome 6, T-lymphocyte receptor genes on chromosomes 7 and 14, and immunoglobulin genes, all of which have been reported to have significant genetic effects on susceptibility to MS (Karpuj et al. 1997; Willer & Ebers, 2000). Further candidate genes include those involved with cytokines, proteolytic enzymes, nitric oxide, myelin precursors, interleukins, interferon, human leukocyte antigen and tumor necrosis factor (Willer & Ebers, 2000).

1.8. Metabolic Disturbances in Multiple Sclerosis

1.8.1. Cell Membrane Lipids

Metabolic disturbances mostly involved in MS are lipid metabolic abnormalities. Lipids are important components of all mammalian cells and have a variety of biological functions, such as the formation of lipid bilayers that provide structural integrity necessary for protein functions, and as an energy reservoir, for example, triglycerides (Caret et al. 1997; Adibhatla & Hatcher, 2007). Membrane lipids consist of phospholipids, into which saturated and unsaturated fatty acids are incorporated, as well as cholesterol. The structures of membrane lipids are extremely diverse, and the functions of neuronal and other membranes depend on the type and composition of phospholipids and cholesterol present, as well as their association with proteins, while the types of fatty acids present in phospholipids are closely correlated with the biological features of the phospholipids (Manzoli et al. 1970; Williams, 1998; Horrobin, 1999).

1.8.1.1. Cell Membrane Phospholipids

All phospholipids (except sphingomyelin) have a 3-carbon glycerol backbone to which two fatty acid molecules and any one of a range of different head-groups are attached. The head-groups (polar groups) may be choline, ethanolamine, inositol or serine (Horrobin, 1999; Koay & Walmsley, 1999). Saturated fatty acids (SATS) and monounsaturated fatty acids (MUFAs) tend to be attached to the Sn1 position, polyunsaturated fatty acids (PUFAs) to the Sn2 position, and the headgroups to the Sn3 position (Horrobin, 1999). Cell membranes are formed by a double layer of phospholipids, with the head-groups of the outer layer facing the extra-cellular spaces, the fatty acids "tails" facing each other, and the head-groups of the inner layer facing the inter-cellular spaces. Choline containing phospholipids, phosphatidylcholine (PC) and sphingomyelin (SM) are mainly on the outer leaflet of plasma membranes, while phosphatidylethanolamine (PE) and phosphatidylserine (PS) are located on the inner leaflet. Phosphatidylcholine is the most abundant phospholipid in animal cell membranes, and PE the second most (Williams, 1998; Barenholz & Thompson, 1999). In the brain however, normal myelin contains a higher percentage of PE than PC, with PE representing about 34 % of the total phospholipids (Manzoli et al. 1970).

The properties of each phospholipid molecule are dependent both upon the type of the head-group and on the nature of the other molecules (fatty acids) attached to the Sn1 and the Sn2 positions (Horrobin, 1999). The fatty acids contained within membrane phospholipids can be saturated (SATS) or mono- and polyunsaturated (MUFAs and PUFAs respectively). Polyunsaturated fatty acids are subdivided into n-9, n-6 and n-3 subtypes (Koay & Walmsley, 1999). Essential fatty acids needed for PUFA synthesis come from the diet, but the body can synthesize both SATS and MUFAs from carbohydrates, if sufficient dietary fat is unavailable (Horrobin, 1999; German & Dillard, 2004). Fatty acids are transported in the blood, either bound to albumin, or in the form of triglycerides (fat) associated with lipoproteins (Horrobin, 1999; Koay & Walmsley, 1999). Fatty acids may be esterified in the form of neutral triglycerides and phospholipids, or non-esterified (free fatty acids) (Koay & Walmsley, 1999). Free fatty acids are the major plasma contributor to brain uptake (Chen et al. 2008).

1.8.1.2. Saturated Fatty Acids

Saturated fatty acids are made of a variable chain length with single carbon-carbon bonds and are straight and rigid (Horrobin, 1999). Both clinical and epidemiological evidence indicates that diets rich in SATS can be harmful to health (German & Dillard, 2004; Zamaria, 2004). However, myelin phospholipids contain a high percentage of SATS and MUFAs, including C16:0 (palmitic acid), C18:0 (stearic acid) and C18:1n-9 (oleic acid) (Manzoli et al. 1970). Furthermore, there is a lack of information about the metabolic aspects of individual dietary SATS (German & Dillard, 2004). A variety of cellular and also viral membrane proteins are modified by fatty acid acylation (Grand, 1989; James & Olson 1990; Okubo et al. 1991). These modifications may play a role in protein targeting and/or signal transduction. C14:0 (myristic acid) and C16:0 (palmitic acid) are metabolites for myristoylation, and palmitoylation respectively. C14:0 is found only in small amounts, while C16:0 is a common metabolite in eukaryotic cells.

Saturated fatty acids have also been shown to display anti-viral and -bacterial properties (Sands, 1977; Cordo et al. 1999; Narasimhan et al. 2006). A series of esters and amides of C14:0 showed in vitro antibacterial activity against gram-positive and gram-negative bacteria which was comparable to that of the standard drug, antibiotic Ciprofloxacin (Narasimhan et al. 2006). Myristic acid analogs have been found to inhibit a late stage in the Junin virus replication cycle (Cordo et al. 1999). Sands (1977) showed that C14:0 and C16:0 did not inactivate enveloped bacteriophage φ6 virus, but did prevent plaque production (Sands, 1977), whereas both C18:1n-9 (oleic acid) and C16:1n-7 (palmitoleic acid) were found to be potent inactivators of the bacteriophage φ6 virus.

Reports on the saturated and monounsaturated fatty acid composition in patients with MS showed that in most studies SATS were increased, while MUFAs were decreased. An increase in SATS, especially C16:0 and C18:0 were found in brain tissue (Chia et al. 1984; Wilson & Tocher, 1991), in plasma (Cherayil, 1984; Cunnane et al. 1989; Holman et al. (1989) and RBCs (Cherayil, 1984; Navarro & Segura, 1989), while a decrease in C20:0 in brain tissue has been reported by Chia et al (1984). A decrease in MUFAs in brain tissue (Chia et al. 1984; Wilson & Tocher, 1991), but an increase in plasma (Holman et al. (1989) was also reported.

1.8.1.3. Unsaturated Fatty Acids

Monounsaturated fatty acids (MUFAs) get their name from the fact that they have one double carbon-carbon bond introduced to the single carbon-carbon bonds of saturated fatty acids. Polyunsaturated fatty acids (PUFAs) have two or more double carbon-carbon bonds (Horrobin, 1999). The double bonds of unsaturated fatty acids are angled and flexible and make the carbon chain more mobile. The more double bonds, the more fluid, flexible and apparently disordered the phospholipid molecule becomes. MUFAs can be synthesized from SATS (Nakamura & Nara, 2004), but PUFAs can only be synthesized from dietary precursors called essential fatty acids (EFAs). The essential fatty acids of the n-6 and n-3 fatty acid series, C18:2n-6 (linoleic acid, LA) and C18:3n-3 (alpha-linolenic acid, ALA) respectively, can not be synthesized in the body and must be ingested from the diet (Roche, 1999; De Pablo & De Cienfuegos, 2000; Zamaria, 2004). The parent dietary n-6 and n-3 essential fatty acids are converted to their fatty acid metabolites (the n-6 and n-3 fatty acid series respectively), by a series of alternating desaturations (addition of a double bond) and elongations (addition of two carbon atoms) (Sprecher, 1982; Horrobin & Manku, 1990). The two series are not inter-convertible (Nightingale et al. 1990; De Pablo & De Cienfuegos 2000). The names of the n-6 and n-3 fatty acids refer to the position of the first double bond in the carbon chain, starting at the methyl end of the molecule (Horrobin, 1999; Koay & Walmsley, 1999). There are three known desaturases in humans: delta-5 (Δ5), delta-6 (Δ6) and delta-9 (Δ9). Delta-6 and delta-5 desaturases are required for the synthesis of PUFAs and highly unsaturated fatty acids (HUFAs) respectively, while delta-9 desaturase catalyze synthesis of MUFAs from SATS. Fatty acids are referred to by an abbreviation of their chemical formulae in the form "Cx:yn-z", where x is the number of carbon atoms (chain lengths), y is the number of double bonds and z is the position of the first double bond, in carbon atoms, from the methyl end of the fatty acid (Nightingale et al. 1990). Some of the metabolic products of C18:2n-6 include C20:3n-6 (dihomo-gamma-linolenic acid, DGLA) and C20:4n-6 (arachidonic acid, AA), while important fatty acids from C18:3n-3 metabolism include C20:5n-3 (eicosapentaenoic acid, EPA) and C22:6n-3 (docosahexaenoic acid, DHA) (Nightingale et al. 1990; Horrobin, 1999; Sprecher, 2000; Pereira et al. 2003).

In contrast to other tissues, there are only small amounts of C18:2n-6 and C18:3n-3 in neuronal phospholipids, but they have large amounts of C20:4n-6 and C22:6n-3, as well as smaller, but important amounts of C20:3n-6, C22:4n-6 (adrenic acid, AdrA), C20:5n-3 and C22:5n-3 (docosapentaenoic acid, DPA) (Horrobin, 1999). C20:4n-6, together with C22:6n-3 forms 80-90 % of the total PUFAs in neuronal and retinal tissue. The human brain has a high demand for C20:4n-6 and C22:4n-6 and requires 4 times the amount of C20:4n-6 than C22:6n-3 on a daily basis (Harbige & Sharief, 2007; Rapoport et al. 2007). The consumption of C20:4n-6 does not significantly change with age (Rapoport et al. 2007). Most neurons need all PUFAs to be preformed (Horrobin, 1999). Plasma C18:2n-6 and C18:3n-3 do not contribute significantly to the brain content of C20:4n-6 or C22:6n-3 respectively (Rapoport et al. 2007), therefore the incorporation of circulating C20:4n-6 and C22:6n-3 into brain tissue represents their rates of consumption by the brain. Glial cells may be involved in these reactions and may supply these fatty acids to neurons (Horrobin, 1999).

1.8.1.3.1. Function of Unsaturated Fatty Acids

Polyunsaturated fatty acids are the basic constituents of phospholipid membranes. They are involved in enzyme and receptor expression, modulation of proteins and cell signaling (Horrobin & Manku, 1990; Horrobin, 1999; De Pablo & De Cienfuegos, 2000; Zamaria, 2004). They also influence membrane fluidity (Nakamura & Nara, 2004), neurotransmission and prostaglandin formation, processes that are vital in the maintenance of normal brain function (Horrobin, 1999; Haag, 2003). Altered lipid metabolism in the cell membrane is believed to be a key event which contributes to CNS injury (Adibhatla et al. 2006; Adibhatla & Hatcher, 2007). Likewise, the fatty acid composition in human immune cells influences their function and can affect phagocytosis, T-lymphocyte signaling and antigen presentation (Calder, 2007). In this, changes in immune cell membrane C20:4n-6, C20:5n-3 and C22:6n-3, the precursors for eicosanoid production, may be important indicators of the pathogenesis of an inflammatory disease.

The PUFA status in blood can be assessed in plasma, platelets, red blood cells and white blood cells (Zamaria, 2004). The plasma fatty acid profile may vary considerably, whereas RBC membrane fatty acids reflect dietary fat intake in relation to the biological half life of these cells (Romon et al. 1995; Zamaria, 2004). RBC membranes, in contrast to other cells, lack the desaturase enzymes and must get their fatty acids from plasma (Allen et al. 2006). Various RBC membrane abnormalities in patients with MS are believed to reflect an altered unsaturated fatty acid content and metabolism (Gul et al. 1970; Homa et al. 1980; Nightingale et al. 1990; Mayer, 1991). Although plasma fatty acids vary considerably, plasma phosphorlipids are also said to reflect changes in PUFAs that occur in tissue phospholipids (Holman et al. 1989). There have been several reports on abnormalities in fatty acid metabolism in cerebral white matter, white blood cells (WBCs), red blood cells (RBCs), platelets and plasma/serum from patients with MS (Baker et al.1964; Cumings et al. 1965; Cherayil, 1984; Fisher et al. 1987; Holman et al. 1989; Navarro & Segura, 1989; Harbige & Sharief, 2007). The disease has been associated with n-3 fatty acid metabolic abnormalities in the CNS, or insufficient dietary intake of these fatty acids (Nightingale et al. 1990). N-6 fatty acids have also been shown to play a role in the pathogenesis and treatment of MS (Harbige & Sharief, 2007).

1.8.1.3.2. Unsaturated Fatty Acids in Brain Tissue

Abnormalities in fatty acid metabolism have been reported, in both apparently normal cerebral white matter and in plaques from MS brain tissue (Boggs & Moscarello, 1980; Chia et al. 1984; Wilson & Tocher, 1991). Myelin is formed from extensions of oligodendrocyte cell membranes. In healthy brains, these membranes have a balanced lipid and protein content (Toshniwal & Zarling, 1992). An increased protein to lipid ratio in the myelin of affected patients has been reported, fully due to a decrease in lipids (Wilson & Tocher, 1991). The protein to lipid ratio showed a 2-fold increase in normal appearing white matter, a 3.3-fold increase in chronic plagues and a 4.3-fold increase in sub-acute plaques in comparison to normal brain tissue. The total myelin yield from normal appearing white matter from patients with MS has been reported to be reduced to two-thirds of that of age-matched control brains (Göpfert et al. 1980).

Increases in C20:4n-6, C22:6n-3 and C20:5n-3 have been reported in the brains from patients with MS (Chia et al. 1984; Wilson & Tocher, 1991), but a reduction in C22:4n-6

(Göpfert et al. 1980) and C22:6n-3 (Kishimoto et al. 1967; Nightingale et al. 1990) in the apparently normal white matter in the CNS of patients with MS have also been reported. The increased C20:4n-6 and C22:6n-3 concentrations reported by Wilson and Tocher (1991) were higher in chronic and sub-acute plaques than in normal appearing white matter. These increases could possibly be due to fatty acids of proliferating and invading astrocytes, which are known to be associated with plaques. However, it is not clear whether the reported alteration in PUFA balance plays a role in the progression of plaques, such as involvement of eicosanoids in disease progression (Horrobin, 1979; Wilson & Tocher, 1991) or whether these changes were entirely secondary to the disease process (Wilson & Tocher, 1991).

Accumulation of free fatty acids (FFAs) in the brains from patients with MS was also reported. Chia et al. (1984) reported slightly higher levels of FFAs in diseased myelin as compared to normal myelin, including increases in FFA C20:4n-6, and Wilson and Tocher (1991) reported increases in total FFAs in plaques. In contrast, Craelius et al. (1981) reported lower FFA C20:4n-6 and FFA C24:4n-6 in diseased white matter. However, the ratio FFA C20:4n-6 to PC C20:4n-6 was higher in the brains from patients with MS than in normal brain tissue, indicating that in MS, FFA C20:4n-6 was released in higher quantities in relation to its phospholipid stock, than in control brains. Glutamate receptors require normal levels of C20:4n-6 in cell membrane phospholipids (Horrobin, 1999), while free fatty acid C20:4n-6 inhibit glutamate uptake into glial cells (Barbour et al. 1989).

1.8.1.3.3. Unsaturated Fatty Acids in Biological Fluids

Baker et al. (1964) reported a decrease in C18:2n-6 in the serum from patients with MS, while Holman et al. (1989) found plasma C18:2n-6 normal, but reported increased levels of C18:3n-6 and subnormal levels of subsequent n-6 fatty acids, including that of C20:4n-6. Cherayil (1984) found reduced C18:2n-6 and C20:4n-6 in plasma from patients with MS. Fisher et al. (1987) found no difference in serum C18:2n-6 between patients with MS and controls. Holman et al. (1989) found the concentration of all n-3 fatty acids to be subnormal in plasma of affected patients, and Cunnane et al. (1989) found the total n-3 fatty acid concentration to be decreased. Cumings et al. (1965) did not find any significant abnormalities in the blood fatty acid profile from patients with MS.

With reagards to RBCs, Cherayil (1984) reported a decrease in C18:2n-6, Navarro and Segura (1989) decreases in both C18:2n-6 and C20:4n-6, Nightingale et al. (1990) an increase in C20:3n-6, while others reported no differences between patients with MS and controls (Evans & Dodd, 1989; Koch et al. 2006). Cunnane et al. (1989) reported metabolic abnormalities between C18:2n-6 and C20:4n-6 in the RBCs from patients with MS. In the n-3 fatty acid series, Nightingale et al. (1990) reported reduced C20:5n-3 levels in patients with MS, but which did not show any relationship with either the EDSS or duration of illness.

Significant decreases in the relative percentages of C18:2n-6 have been shown in peripheral blood lymphocyte (PBL) membranes from patients with MS, with accompanying lower plasma levels (Tsang et al. 1976; Cherayil, 1984), while Fisher et al. (1987) showed a similar decrease in C18:2n-6 in the white blood cells and platelets from patients with MS, but not in their serum. Harbige and Sharief (2007) reported C20:3n-6 and C20:4n-6 to be lower in peripheral blood mononuclear cell (PBMC) membranes in 20-30 percent of the patients studied. They also demonstrated a disturbed metabolic relationship between C18:2n-6 and C20:3n-6, as well as between C20:3n-6 and C20:4n-6, in the PBMC membranes from patients with MS, as compared to healthy controls. Fatty acid metabolic abnormalities in cell membranes could indicate a problem with desaturases, or greater requirement for C20:4n-6 in the group of patients studied. Abnormalities in the relationship between plasma and cell membrane fatty acids from patients with MS reported by Navarro and Segura (1989), suggested a relative deficiency of essential fatty acids (Navarro & Segura, 1989).

1.8.1.4. Cell Membrane Cholesterol

Cholesterol, a common steroid, is found in the membranes of most animal cells, and is involved in the regulation of membrane barrier properties, such as membrane fluidity and permeability (Voet & Voet, 1995; Caret et al. 1997; Barenholz, 2002). The fused ring system of cholesterol provides it with greater rigidity than other membrane lipids, reducing membrane fluidity and permeability (Mouritsen & Jorgensen, 1994; Voet & Voet, 1995; Mouritsen & Jorgensen, 1998; Mitchell & Litman, 2001; Barenholz, 2002). Wilson and Tocher (1991) reported the percentage cholesterol to be generally lower in MS plaques, but the differences were not significant. Chia et al. (1984) and Boggs and Moscarello (1980) did not find the cholesterol to phospholipid ratio in myelin different from that of normal myelin.

1.8.2. Cell Membrane Fluidity

Because phospholipids make up the structure of biological membranes, they can be used to evaluate membrane integrity. Phospholipids have different headgroups, PC, PE, PS, PI and SM, and because these differ in function and structure, their composition will determine how closely they can pack together in the cell membrane, and therefore how rigid or fluid the membrane structure will be. Cell membrane lipids may be more ordered (closely packed) or less ordered (less packed) (Williams, 1998). Phospholipids with smaller head-groups such as PE, will pack closer together than those with bigger head-groups, such as PC. In addition, because the phospholipids contain fatty acids with different chain lengths and different degrees of unsaturation, these will have a modulating effect on the way membrane phospholipids can pack (Williams, 1998). Phospholipids with increased saturated (SATS) concentrations, which contain no double bonds, and monounsaturated (MUFAs), which contain one double bond, will therefore pack closer together than phospholipids with increased polyunsaturated (PUFA) concentrations, which contain two or more double bonds. The double bonds of MUFAs and PUFAs are angled and flexible and make the carbon chain more mobile, which prevent close packing. An increase in the number of double bonds will therefore result in a more fluid and apparently disordered membrane structure (Horrobin, 1999). The concentration of cholesterol present in the membrane will further determine membrane fluidity (Voet & Voet, 1995; Mouritsen & Jorgensen, 1998; Barenholz, 2002).

The composition of membrane phospholipids, their fatty acids and cholesterol specify the degree of membrane permeability and fluidity, which have an effect on imbedded protein interactions and membrane-bound enzyme and receptor expression (Mouritsen & Jorgensen, 1994; Voet & Voet, 1995; Mouritsen & Jorgensen, 1998; Williams, 1998; De Pablo & De Cienfuegos, 2000; Mitchell & Litman, 2001; Barenholz, 2002; Zamaria, 2004). In this, organisms have the ability to adjust the order or fluidity of their cellular membranes to optimize interaction with their physiochemical environment (Williams, 1998). However, there are changes in either the cell membrane composition itself, or induced from the environment, such as changes in temperature and pressure, that may impair membrane structure and function, and may even result in cell death.

1.8.2.1 Measurement of Cell Membrane Fluidity

Various methods, such as electron spin resonance (ESR) (Boggs & Moscarello, 1980; Kurantsin-Mills et al. 1982), fluorescence polarization spectroscopy (Boggs & Moscarello, 1980) and microfiltration (Pollock et al. 1982) have been used to investigate membrane fluidity in patients with MS. No difference was found between MS patients and controls in membrane fluidity (Boggs & Moscarello, 1980; Kurantsin-Mills et al. 1982) or RBC deformability (Pollock et al. 1982). Chia et al. (1984) used x-ray diffraction studies to investigate myelin from both healthy controls and MS patients. They found that at 25 °C, tissue from both normal and MS brains contained a mixture of liquid-crystalline-phase lipids and ordered-crystalline-phase lipids, as in normal subjects. Lipids in the liquid-crystalline-phase is in a fluid-phase, while lipids in the ordered-crystalline-phase is in a gel-phase and have close hexagonal packing of the hydrocarbon chain, that is the fatty acid tails are packed closely together. When these results were repeated at 50 °C, the authors found that myelin from MS patients contained liquid-crystalline-phase lipids only, while normal myelin still contained both liquid-crystalline-phase lipids and ordered-crystalline-phase lipids. These results suggested some abnormality in the lipid composition in myelin from MS patients.

The liquid-crystalline-phase lipids and ordered-crystalline-phase lipids reported by Chia et al. (1984), form lamellar and hexagonal structures respectively, of which the lamellar phase is dominant (Harlos & Eibl, 1981). Cell membrane fluidity is regulated by variation of the ratio of liquid-crystalline-phase lipids to ordered-crystalline-phase lipids in the membrane. A transition from the liquid-crystalline-phase (lamellar phase) to an ordered-crystalline-phase (hexagonal phase) only, will result in a non-functional membrane (Harlos & Eibl, 1981; Chia et al. 1984; Williams, 1998). At the other extreme, membrane order can also become steadily decreased and may undergo another phase transition, to the reversed-hexagonal phase, which is also non-lamellar, and in which the phospholipid molecules are in total disarray (Williams, 1998). Membrane function can however be impaired long before either of these transition points is reached (Williams, 1998). The ratio of ordered-crystalline-phase lipids to liquid-crystalline-phase lipids in the membrane corresponds to phospholipid PE to PC ratio (Williams, 1998).

Membrane lipids differ in their head-groups and hydrocarbon chains, and have therefore been used to investigate the degree of fluidity of membranes as well. Formulae that have been used to calculate membrane fluidity include the following: the membrane saturated nature as measured by the phospholipid PC + SM/PE + PS ratio (Allen et al. 2006), membrane fluidity and permeability as measured by the cholesterol to phospholipid ratio, the membrane ordered-crystalline-phase lipids to liquid-crystalline-phase lipids as measured by the phospholipid PE to PC ratio, as well as the rheologic properties (deformability) of RBCs, as measured by the phospholipid PE to PS ratio (Labrouche et al. 1996; Allen et al. 2006). RBCs can loose their flexibility due to changes in the cell membrane lipid composition and become rigid (Allen et al. 2006). Decreased deformability can make oxygen delivery through the capillaries difficult. Furthermore, RBCs with decreased deformability are known to respond to PGE2, and the sensitivity of these cells to PGE2 suggests that RBCs may be a primary target for prostaglandin action (Allen and Rasmussen, 1971; Harris et al. 2001). The membrane SATS to PUFA ratio has also been used as an indication of membrane fluidity (Candiloros et al. 1996; Allen et al. 2006).

No differences were reported in membrane cholesterol concentrations or in the relationship between membrane cholesterol and phospholipids between patients with MS and control subjects (Boggs & Moscarello, 1980; Chia et al. 1984). However, decreases in plasma and/or RBC membrane PUFAs were reported to be replaced by increases in SATS and/or MUFAs (Cherayil, 1984; Cunnane et al. 1989; Holman et al. 1989; Navarro & Segura, 1989; Nightingale et al. 1990). If essential fatty acids (PUFAs) are unavailable, they will be replaced by the nonessential fatty acids, SATS and MUFAs (Horrobin, 1999). Reports on the fatty acid composition of the brain from patients with MS did not show this trend. A decrease in PUFAs was reported (Göpfert et al. 1980), but increases were also reported (Chia et al. 1984; Wilson & Tocher, 1991). Increases in individual SATS were reported (Chia et al. 1984; Wilson & Tocher, 1991), but decreases in others were also reported (Chia et al. 1984). In general, decreases were found in MUFAs (Göpfert et al. 1980; Chia et al. 1984; Wilson & Tocher, 1991).

1.8.3 Lipids as Mediators of Inflammation

Although the reports are inconsistent, particularly C18:2n-6 (linoleic acid, LA) and C20:4n-6 have been shown to be reduced in the plasma, platelets, RBCs, WBCs, and CSF from patients with MS (Harbige & Sharief, 2007). Harbige and Sharief (2007) reported that together with the loss of C18:2n-6 and C20:4n-6 from PBMC membranes, an increase was shown in the production of pro-inflammatory cytokines TNF-α and interleukin-1beta (IL-1β), and a decrease in anti-inflammatory transforming growth factor beta (TGF-β). These results suggested that the loss of C18:2n-6 and C20:4n-6 in PBMC membranes from patients with MS was due to the inflammatory process. These fatty acids are precursors for eicosanoid production, which are reported to be increased during the inflammatory response in neurodegenerative diseases (De Pablo & De Cienfuegos, 2000; Tilley et al. 2001; Farooqui et al. 2007; Khanapure et al. 2007). Because of the relatively high amount of C20:4n-6 in immune cell membrane phospholipids, it is typically the major precursor for eicosanoid synthesis e.g. prostaglandin E2 (PGE2) and leukotriene B4 (LTB4) (Calder, 2007). Inflammatory activation of the enzyme phospholipase A2 (PLA2) leads to the release of C20:4n-6 from cell membrane phospholipids, which in turn is metabolized by cyclooxygenases (COX), yielding eicosanoids (Herschman, 1996; Calder, 2001; Simopoulos, 2002; Bagga et al. 2003; Gilroy et al. 2004; Farooqui et al. 2007). An increase in PLA2 activity is associated with neurological disorders such as MS (Farooqui et al. 2007).

Eicosanoids regulate cellular functions, but their effects also depend on each precursor fatty acid and the cell type concerned (Horrobin & Manku, 1990; De Pablo & De Cienfuegos, 2000; Zamaria, 2004). Prostaglandin H2 (PGH2) is produced by both COX isoforms (COX1 and COX2), and is the common substrate for a series of specific synthase enzymes that produce prostaglandin D2 (PGD2), PGE2, prostaglandin F2α (PGF2α), prostaglandin I2 (PGI2) and thromboxane A2 (TXA2) (Tilley et al. 2001). Mast cells and neutrophils generate predominantly PGD2, while monocytes and macrophages produce PGE2 and TXA2 (Tilley et al. 2001; Calder, 2007). This profile will change according to the different stages of the immune response (Calder, 2007). In resting macrophages, TXA2 is produced in excess of PGE2, while this ratio changes in favor of PGE2 production after an immune response is elicited (Tilley et al. 2001). In the brain, the proportion of C20:4n-6 lost to metabolic processes, such as eicosanoid production, is replaced by FFAs from the plasma (Chen et al. 2008).

PGE2 is highly pro-inflammatory (Simopoulos, 2002; Bagga et al. 2003; Haag, 2003), while prostaglandin E1 (PGE1), derived from the metabolism of C20:3n-6 (dihomo-gamma-linolenic acid, DGLA), is considered to have intermediate properties (Horrobin & Manku, 1990; Haag, 2003). In contrast, prostaglandins derived from the metabolism of the n-3 PUFAs, show anti-inflammatory effects (Grimm et al. 2002; Culp et al. 1979; Simopoulos, 2002; Bagga et al. 2003; Calder, 2007). C20:5n-3 is metabolized to prostaglandin E3 (PGE3), which has anti-inflammatory properties (Hansen, 1983; Bagga et al. 2003; Haag, 2003; Zamaria, 2004). C22:6n-3 is metabolized to docosanoids (Farooqui et al. 2007; Chen et al. 2008), which include resolvins, docosatrienes and protectins (Farooqui et al. 2007), and which are anti-inflammatory in nature (Nakamura & Nara, 2004; Calder, 2007; Farooqui et al. 2007).

Altered prostaglandin production is associated with a variety of illnesses, including inflammation (Herschman, 1996; Bagga et al. 2003). The amplification of PGE2 may be active in brain pathologies such as MS (Repovic et al. 2003). In this regard, Hofman et al. (1986) found immune cells in MS lesions that exhibited positive staining for prostaglandin E (PGE), which was not found in normal brain tissue. The presence of stimulated cells present in the brains of patients with MS suggested an active immune mechanism in the pathogenesis of MS. Prostaglandins are very short-lived substances, and measurements of the levels of eicosanoids in body fluids are difficult (Horrobin & Manku, 1990). Evaluating their fatty acid precursors could however give an indication of an abnormal metabolism.

Conclusion

Membrane fatty acid metabolic abnormalities have been reported in MS and have been linked to the pathogenesis of the disease. Reports are inconsistent, but a reduction in both n-6 and n-3 polyunsaturated fatty acids (PUFAs), with an increase in saturated fatty acids (SATS) and monounsaturated fatty acids (MUFAs), has been reported. In particular, a reduction in the n-6 fatty acids, C18:2n-6 and its elongation product, C20:4n-6 have consistently been reported in the plasma and cell membranes from patients with MS. Both phospholipase A2 (PLA2) activity and prostaglandin E2 (PGE2) production is known to be increased during inflammatory activation. PLA2 releases C20:4n-6 from membrane phospholipids, making the free fatty acids (FFAs) available for PGE2 synthesis. In this regard, the released FFA C20:4n-6 itself is known to be toxic to surrounding cells, and would therefore add to the effects of a possibly increased pro-inflammatory PGE2 concentration. Because of the relatively high amount of C20:4n-6 in immune cell membrane phospholipids, eicosanoids synthesized from C20:4n-6, such as PGE2, are known to be produced in increased amounts upon stimulation. Results reported by Harbige and Sharief (2007), who showed an increase in pro-inflammatory cytokines with a decrease in PBMC membrane C20:4n-6, suggested that a decrease in membrane C20:4n-6 could be indicative of pro-inflammatory effects. In this regard, synthesis of both pro-inflammatory cytokines and pro-inflammatory prostaglandins are known to be upregulated during inflammation. Furthermore, RBC membranes with diminished fluidity are vulnerable to hydrolysis by secretory PLA2 (sPLA2) (Harris et al. 2001), and RBC membrane fluidity as measured by the increase in the SATS to PUFA ratio in patients with MS has been reported to be decreased (higher rigidity) (Hon et al. 2009a), suggesting that in patients with MS RBC membranes could be vulnerable to sPLA2 activity.

Inflammatory responses usually result in self-limiting healing processes, but increased immune cell activity has been reported in the CNS from patients with MS. Microglia are the main mediators of neuro-inflammation and also initiate recruitment of leukocytes from the blood stream into brain tissue. Glial cells have been shown to be involved in CNS disorders, especially in MS. They precede other immune cells such as T-lymphocytes, differentiated B-lymphocytes and early activated macrophages in apoptotic zones. Leukocytes are not present in healthy brains, and therefore increased immune cell activity in the brain could change the fatty acid requirements of brain tissue from patients with MS, and could possibly deplete sources elsewhere, such as from compromised RBC membranes. The amplification of PGE2 may be active in brain pathologies such as MS (Repovic et al. 2003) and Hofman et al. (1986) reported immune cells from MS brain lesions which stained positive for prostaglandin E (PGE), which was not found in normal brain tissue. These reductions in membrane fatty acids could contribute to the pathogenesis of the disease, both through depletion of membrane fatty acid concentrations, and possibly by an excess of eicosanoids.

Membrane fatty acid concentrations were reported to correlate with disease outcome as measured by the Kurtzke Expanded Disability Status Scale and its Functional System Scores (EDSS and FSS respectively) (Hon et al. 2009b; 2009c). RBC membrane C20:4n-6 showed inverse correlations with the EDSS and FSS (Hon et al. 2009b), and PBMC membrane C20:4n-6 with the FSS (Hon et al. 2009c), linking decreased membrane C20:4n-6 directly to the pathogenesis of the disease. Whether this relationship is due to impairment of the RBC membrane and therefore diminished ability to deliver oxygen to the brain and other tissue, and/or because of an indication of increased eicosanoid production, is not clear, and needs further investigation.

In MS, decreases in plasma and/or membrane PUFAs were reported to be replaced by increases in SATS and/or MUFAs. Diets rich in SATS can be harmful to health and is generally associated with the development of many diseases, including MS (Van Meeteren et al. 2005). However, there is lack of information about the individual dietary SATS (German & Dillard, 2004). Specific membrane SATS have been identified that in MS patients at least, were found to be associated with a worse outcome, which were the longer-chain saturated fatty acids, while the shorter-chain saturated fatty acids, including C14:0 and C16:0, metabolites for myristoylation, and palmitoylation respectively, correlated with a better disease outcome as measured by the EDSS and FSS (Hon et al. 2009d).

Changes in membrane lipid composition can be expected to have an effect on membrane structure and function. The composition of membrane phospholipids, their fatty acids and cholesterol specify the degree of membrane rigidity, permeability and fluidity. An altered fatty acid profile would result in changes in membrane fluidity as measured by the relationship between membrane lipids. Lower RBC membrane fluidity (higher rigidity) as measured by the SATS to PUFA ratio was observed in patients with MS and which were reported to be closely interrelated with inflammation and disease outcome in patients with MS (Hon et al. 2009a).

In conclusion therefore, the changes in C20:4n-6 concentration in blood cell membranes from patients with MS is important in the pathogenesis of the disease. In addition, that in the presence of uncontrolled inflammation such as in MS, altered fatty acid composition indirectly compromises the cell membrane structure and function, and thereby contributes to the disease progression.

References

Aboul-Enein, F., Rauschka, H., Kornek, B., Stadelmann, C., Stefferl, A., Brück, W., Lucchinetti, C., Schmidbauer, M., Jellinger, K. & Lassmann, H. (2003). Preferential loss of myelin-associated glycoprotein reflects hypoxia-like white matter damage in stroke and inflammatory brain diseases. *J Neuropathol Exp Neurol,* 62:25-33.

Adam, P., Sobek, O., Taborsky, L. Hildebrand, T., Tutterova, O. & Zacek, P. (2003). CSF and serum orosomucoid (α-1-acid glycoprotein) in patients with multiple sclerosis: a comparison among particular subgroups of MS patients. *Clin Chim Acta, 334*:107-110.

Adibhatla, R.M. & Hatcher, J.F. (2007). Role of lipids in brain injury and diseases. *Future Lipidol,* 2:403-422.

Allen, H.G., Allen, J.C., Boyd, L.C., Alston-Mills, B.P. & Fenner, G.P. (2006). Determination of membrane lipid differences in insulin resistant diabetes mellitus type 2 in whites and blacks. *Nutrition,* 22:1096-1102.

Allen, J.E. & Rasmussen, H. (1971). Human Red Blood Cells: Prostaglandin E_2, Epinephrine, and Isoproterenol Alter Deformability. *Science,* 174:512-514.

Antonovsky, A., Leibowitz, U., Smith, H.A., Medalie, J.M., Balogh, M., Kats, R., Halpern, L. & Alter, M. (1965). Epidemiologic study of multiple sclerosis in Israel. *Arch Neurol,* 13:183-193.

Antony, J.M., Van Marle, G., Opii, W., Butterfield, D.A., Mallet, F., Yong, V.W., Wallace, J.L., Deacon, R.M., Warren, K. & Power, C. (2004). Human endogenous retrovirus glycoprotein-mediated induction of redox reactants causes oligodendrocyte death and demyelination. *Nat Neurosci,* 7:1088-1095.

Bagga, D., Wang, L., Farias-Eisner, R., Glaspy, J.A. & Reddy, S.T. (2003). Differential effects of prostaglandin derived from ω-6 and ω-3 polyunsaturated fatty acids on COX-2 expression and IL-6 secretion. *PNAS,* 100:1751-1756.

Baker, R.W.R., Thompson, R.H.S. & Zilkha, K.J. (1964). Serum fatty acids in multiple sclerosis. *J Neurol Neurosurg Psychiatry,* 27:408-414.

Barbour, B., Szatkowski, M. Ingledew, N. & Attwell, D. (1989). Arachidonic acid induces prolonged inhibition of glutamate uptake into glial cells, *Nature,* 342:918-920.

Barenholz, Y. & Thompson, T.E. (1999). Sphingomyelin: biophysical aspects. *Chem Phys Lipids,* 102:29-34.

Barenholz, Y. (2002). Cholesterol and other membrane active sterols: from membrane evolution to "rafts". *Prog Lipid Res,* 41:1-5.

Barnett, M.H. & Prineas, J.W. (2004). Relapsing and remitting multiple sclerosis: pathology of the newly forming lesion. *Ann Neurol,* 55:458-68.

Bates, D., Fawcett, P.R.W., Shaw, D.A. & Weightman, D. (1978). Polyunsaturated fatty acids in treatment of acute remitting multiple sclerosis. *BMJ,* 2:1390-1391.

Bjartmar, C. & Trapp, B. D. (2001). Axonal and neuronal degeneration in multiple sclerosis: mechanisms and functional consequences. *Curr Opin Neurol,* 14:271-278.

Boggs, J.M. & Moscarello, M.A, (1980). A comparison of composition and fluidity of multiple sclerosis and normal myelin, *Neurochem Res,* 5:319-336.

Brown, KA. (2001). Factors modifying the migration of lymphocytes across the blood-brain barrier. *Int Immunopharmacol,* 1:2043-2062.

Brück, W. (2005). Clinical implications of neuropathological findings in multiple sclerosis. *J Neurol,* 252:III/10 - III/14.

Butcher, P.J. 1986. Milk consumption and multiple sclerosis – an etiological hypothesis. *Med Hypotheses,* 19:169-178.

Calder, P.C. (2001). Polyunsaturated fatty acids, inflammation, and immunity. *Lipids*, 36: 1007-1024.

Calder, P.C. (2007). Immunomodulation by omega-3 fatty acids. *Prostaglandins Leukot Essent Fatty Acids,* 77:327-335.

Candiloros, H., Zeghari, N., Ziegler, O., Donner, M. & Drouin, P. (1996). Hyperinsulinemia is related to erythrocyte phospholipid composition and membrane fluidity changes in obese nondiabetic women. *J Clin Endocrinol Metab,* 81:2912-2918.

Caret, R.L., Denniston, K.J. & Topping, J.J. (1997). Lipids and their functions in biochemical systems. In Wheatley, C.H. (ed). *Principles and applications of inorganic, organic and biological chemistry.* 2nd ed. Boston: McGraw-Hill: 379-407.

Cendrowski, W., Wender, M., Dominik, W., Flejsierowicz, Z., Owsianowski, M. & Popiel, M. (1969). Epidemiological study of multiple sclerosis in Western Poland. *Eur Neurol,* 2:90-108.

Chatzimanolis, N., Kraus, J. Bauer, R. Engelhardt, B. Bregenzer, T., Kuehne, B.S., Tofighi, J., Laske, C., Stolz, E., Blaes, F., Voigt, K., Traupe, H., Kaps, M. & Oschmann, P. (2004). CD45RA + ICAM-3 + lymphocytes in interferon-β1b-treated and –untreated patients with relapsing-remitting multiple sclerosis. *Acta Neurol Scand,* 110: 377-385.

Chen, C.T., Green, J.T., Orr, S.K. & Bazinet, R.P. (2008). *Regulation of brain polyunsaturated fatty acid uptake and turnover.* Prostaglandins Leukot Essent Fatty Acids, 79:85-91.

Cherayil, G.D. (1984). Sialic acid and fatty acid concentrations in lymphocytes, red blood cells and plasma from patients with multiple sclerosis. *J Neurol Sci,* 63:1-10.

Chia, L.S., Thompson, J.E. & Moscarello, M.A. (1984). Alteration of lipid-phase behavior in multiple sclerosis myelin revealed by wide-angle x-ray diffraction. *Proc Natl Acad Sci* USA, 81:1871-1874.

Chwastiak, L., Ehde, D.M., Gibbons, L.E., Sullivan, M., Bowen, J.D. & Kraft, G.H. (2002). Depressive symptoms and severity of illness in multiple sclerosis: Epidemiologic study of a large community sample. *Am J Psychiatry,* 159:1862-1868.

Compston, A. & Coles, A. (2002). Multiple sclerosis. *Lancet*, 359:1221–1231.

Cooper, R.L.T. (1997). Multiple Scleosis: an immune legacy? *Med Hypotheses,* 49:307-311.

Cordo, S.M., Candurra, N.A. & Damonte, E.B. (1999). Myristic acid analogs are inhibitors of Junin virus replication. *Microb Infect,* 1:609-614.

Craelius, W., Gurmankin, R.S., Rosenheck, D.M. & Schaefer, D.C. (1981). Free fatty acid patterns in normal and multiple sclerosis white matter. *Acta Neurol Scand,* 63:197-203.

Culp, B.R., Titus, B.G. & Lands, W.E. (1979). Inhibition of prostaglandins by eicosapentaenoic acid. *Prostag Med,* 3:269-278.

Cumings, J.N., Shortman, R.C. & Skrbic, T. (1965). Lipid studies in the blood and brain in multiple sclerosis and motor neurone disease. *J Clin Pathol,* 18:641-644.

Cunnane, S.C., Ho, S-Y., Dore-Duffy, P., Ells, K.R. & Horrobin, D.F. (1989). Essential fatty acid and lipid profiles in plasma and erythrocytes in patients with multiple sclerosis. *Am J Clin Nutr,* 50:801-806.

De Pablo, M.A. & De Cienfuegos, G.Á. (2000). Modulatory effects of dietary lipids on immune system functions. *Immunol Cell Biol,* 78:31-39.

De Villiers, J.N.P, Treurnicht, F.K., Warnich, L. Carr, J., Van Rensburg, S.J. & Kotze, M.J. (2006). Analysis of viral and genetic factors in South African patients with multiple sclerosis. *Metab Brain Dis,* 21:163-169.

Evans, P. & Dodd, G. (1989). Erythrocyte fatty acids in multiple sclerosis. *Acta Neurol Scand, 80*:501-503.

Farinotti, M., Simi, S., Di Pietrantonj, C., McDowell, N., Brait, L., Lupo, D. & Filippini, G. (2007). Dietary interventions for multiple sclerosis. *Cochrane Database Syst Rev,* (1) CD004192.

Farooqui, A.A., Horrocks, L.A. & Farooqui, T. (2007). Modulation of inflammation in brain: a matter of fat. *J Neurochem,* 101:577-599.

Fassas, A., Anagnostopoulos, A., Kazis, A., Kapinas, K., Sakellari, I., Kimiskidis, V., Smias, C., Eleftheriadis, N. & Tsimourtou, V. (2000). Autologous stem cell transplantation in progressive multiple sclerosis--an interim analysis of efficacy. *J Clin Immunol,* 20:24-30.

Fassas, A., Passweg, J.R., Anagnostopoulos, A., Kazis, A., Kozak, T., Havrdova, E., Carreras, E., Graus, F., Kashyap, A., Openshaw, H., Schipperus, M., Deconinck, E., Mancardi, G., Marmont, A., Hansz, J., Rabusin, M., Zuazu Nagore, F.J., Besalduch, J., Dentamaro, T., Fouillard, L., Hertenstein, B., La Nasa, G., Musso, M., Papineschi, F., Rowe, J.M., Saccardi, R., Steck, A., Kappos, L., Gratwohl, A., Tyndall, A. & Samijn, J.; Autoimmune Disease Working Party of the European Group for Blood and Marrow Transplantation. (2002). Hematopoietic stem cell transplantation for multiple sclerosis. A retrospective multicenter study. *J Neurol,* 249:1088-1097.

Fisher, M., Johnson, M.H., Natale, A.M. & Levine, P.H. (1987). Linoleic acid levels in white blood cells, platelets, and serum of multiple sclerosis patients. *Acta Neurol Scand,* 76:241-245.

Gay, F.W., Drye, T.J., Dick, G.W. A. & Esiri, M.M. (1997). The application of multifactorial cluster analysis in the staging of plaques in early multiple sclerosis. Identification and characterization of the primary demylinating lesion. *Brain,* 120:1461-1483.

German, J.B. & Dillard, C.J. (2004). Saturated fats: what dietary intake? *Am J Clin Nutr,* 80:550-559.

Gilroy, D.W., Newson, J., Sawmynaden, P., Willoughby, D.A. & Croxtall, J.D. (2004). A novel role for phospholipase A2 isoforms in the checkpoint control of acute inflammation. *FASEB J,* 18:489-498.

Giovannoni, G., Miller, D.H., Losseff, N.A., Sailer, M., Lewellyn-Smith, N., Thompson, A.J. & Thompson, E.J. (2001). Serum inflammatory markers and clinical/MRI markers of disease progression in multiple sclerosis. *J Neurol, 248*:487-495.

Giovannoni, G., Thorpe, J.W., Kidd, D., Kendall, B.E., Moseley, I.F., Thompson, A.J., Keir, G., Miller, D.H., Feldmann, M. & Thompson, E.J. (1996). Soluble E-selectin in multiple sclerosis: raised concentrations in patients with primary progressive disease. *J Neurol Neurosurg Psychiatry,* 60:20-26.

Göpfert, E., Pytlik, S. & Debuch, H. (1980). 2′,3′ -Cyclic nucleotide 3′ -Phosphohydrolase and lipids of myelin from multiple sclerosis and normal brains. *J Neurochem,* 34:732-739.

Grand, R.J.A. (1989). Acylation of viral and eukaryotic proteins. *Biochemistry,* 258:625-638.

Grimm, H., Mayer, K., Mayser, P. & Eigenbrodt, E. (2002). Regulatory potential of n-3 fatty acids in immunological and inflammatory processes. *Br J Nutr,* 87:S59-S67.

Gul, S., Smith, A.D., Thompson, R.H.S., Wright, H.P. & Zilkha, K.J. (1970). Fatty acid composition of phospholipids from platelets and erythrocytes in multiple sclerosis. *J Neurol Neurosurg Psychiatry,* 33:506-510.

Haag, M. (2003). Essential fatty acids and the brain. *Can J Psychiatry,* 48:195-203.

Hafler, D.A. (2004). Multiple sclerosis. *J Clin Invest,* 113:788-794.

Hansen, H.S. (1983). Dietary essential fatty acids and in vivo prostaglandin production in mammals. *World Rev Nutr Diet,* 42:102-134.

Harbige, L.S. & Sharief, M.K. (2007). Polyunsaturated fatty acids in the pathogenesis and treatment of multiple sclerosis. *Br J Nutr,* 98:S46-S53.

Harlos, K. & Eibl, H. (1981). Hexagonal phases in phospholipids with saturated chains: Phosphatidylethanolamines and phosphatidic acids. *Biochemistry,* 20:2888-2892.

Harris, F.M., Smith, S.K. & Bell, J.D. (2001). Physical Properties of Erythrocyte Ghosts That Determine Susceptibility to Secretory Phospholipase A_2. *J Biol Chem,* 276:22722-22731

Henry, O.F., Blacher, J., Verdavaine, J., Duviquet, M. & Safar, M.E. (2003). Alpha 1-acid glycoprotein is an independent predictor of in-hospital death in the elderly. *Age Aging,* 32:37-42.

Herschman, H.R. (1996). Prostaglandin synthase 2. Biochim Biophys Acta, 1299:125-140.

Hofman, F.M., Von Hanwehr, R.I., Dinarello, C.A., Mizel, S.B., Hinton, D. & Merrill, J.E. (1986). Immunoregulatory molecules and IL-2 receptors identified in multiple sclerosis brain, *J Immunol,* 136:3239-3245.

Holman, R.T., Johnson, S.B. & Kokmen, E. (1989). Deficiencies of polyunsaturated fatty acids and replacement by nonessential fatty acids in plasma lipids in multiple sclerosis. *Proc Natl Acad Sci* USA, 86:4720-4724.

Homa, S.T., Belin, J., Smith, A.D., Monro, J.A. & Zilkha, K.J. (1980). Levels of linoleate and arachidonate in red blood cells of healthy individuals and patients with multiple sclerosis. *J Neurol Neurosurg Psychiatry,* 43:106-110.

Hon, G., Hassan, M., van Rensburg, S.J., Abel, S., Marais, D.W., van Jaarsveld, P., Smuts, C., Henning, F. Erasmus, R., & Matsha, T. (2009c). Immune cell membrane fatty acids and inflammatory marker, C-reactive protein, in patients with multiple sclerosis. *Br J Nutr,* 102:1334-1340.

Hon, G.M, Hassan, M.S., van Rensburg, S.J., Abel, S., Marais, D.W., van Jaarsveld, P., Smuts, C.M., Henning, F., Erasmus, R.T. & Matsha, T. (2009b). Erythrocyte membrane fatty acids in patients with multiple sclerosis. *Mult Scler,* 15:759-762.

Hon, G.M., Hassan, M.S., Van Rensburg, S.J, Abel, S., Van Jaarsveld, P., Erasmus, R.T. & Matsha, T. (2009a). Red blood cell membrane fluidity in the etiology of multiple sclerosis. *J Membrane Biol,* 232:25-34, DOI 10.1007/s00232-009-9213-1.

Hon, G.M., Hassan, M.S., Van Rensburg, S.J., Abel, S., Erasmus, R.T. & Matsha, T. (2009d). Membrane saturated fatty acids and disease progression in Multiple Sclerosis patients. *Metab Brain Dis,* 24:561-568, DOI 10.1007/s11011-009-9159-0.

Horrobin, D.F. & Manku, M.S. (1990). Clinical biochemistry of essential fatty acids. In Horrobin, D.F. (ed). Omega-6 essential fatty acids. *Pathophysiology and roles in clinical medicine.* New York: Alan R. Liss Inc: 21-49.

Horrobin, D.F. (1979). Multiple sclerosis: the rational basis for treatment with colchicine and evening primrose oil. *Med Hypotheses,* 5:365-378.

Horrobin, D.F. (1999). The phospholipid concept of psychiatric disorders and its relationship to the neurodevelopmental concept of schizophrenia. In Peet, M., Glen, I. & Horrobin, D.F. (eds). *Phospholipid spectrum disorder in psychiatry.* Lancashire, UK: Marius Press: 3-16.

Hunter, S.F. & Hafler, D.A. (2000). Ubiquitous pathogens. Links between infection and autoimmunity in MS? *Neurology,* 55:164-165.

James, G. & Olson, E.N. (1990). Fatty acylated proteins as components of intracellular signaling pathways. *Biochemistry,* 29:2623-2623.

Jelinek, G. (2000). *Taking control of multiple sclerosis. Natural and medical therapies to prevent its progression.* 2nd ed. Victoria, Australia: Hyland House Publishing Pty Ltd: 28-30.

Karpuj, M.V., Steinman, L. & Oksenberg, J.R. (1997). Multiple sclerosis: a polygenic disease involving epistatic interactions, germline rearrangements and environmental effects. *Neurogenetics,* 1:21-28.

Khanapure, S.P., Garvey, D.S., Janero, D.R. & Letts, L.G. (2007). Eicosanoids in inflammation: Biosynthesis, pharmacology and therapeutic frontiers. *Curr Top Med Chem,* 7:311-340.

Kishimoto, Y., Radin, N.S., Tourtelotte, W.W., Parker, J.A. & Itabashi, H.H. (1967). Gangliosis and glycerophosphates in multiple sclerosis white matter. *Arch Neurol,* 16:44-54.

Koay, E.S.C. & Walmsley, N. (1996). *Plasma lipids and lipoproteins. A primer of Chemical Pathology*. Singapore: World Scientific: 191-211.

Koch, M., Ramsaransing, G.S.M., Fokkema, M.R., Heersema, D.J. & De Keyser, J. (2006). Erythrocyte membrane fatty acids in benign and progressive forms of multiple sclerosis. *J Neurol Sci,* 244:123-126.

Kulmatycki, K.M. & Jamali, F. (2006). Drug disease interactions: Role of inflammatory mediators in depression and variability in antidepressant drug response. *J Pharm Pharmaceut Sci,* 9:292-306.

Kurantsin-Mills, J., Samji, N., Moscarello, M.A. & Boggs, J.M. (1982). Comparison of membrane structure, osmotic fragility, and morphology of multiple sclerosis and normal erythrocytes. *Neurochem Res,* 7:1523-1540.

Kurtzke, J.F. (1983). Rating neurologic impairment in multiple sclerosis: an expanded disability status scale (EDSS). *Neurology,* 33:1444-1452.

Labrouche, S., Freyburger, G., Gin H., Boisseau, M.R. & Cassagne, C. (1996). Changes in phospholipid composition of blood cell membranes (erythrocyte, platelet, and polymorphonuclear) in different types of diabetes- clinical and biological correlations. *Metabolism,* 45:57-71.

Lassmann, H., Brück, W. & Lucchinettii, C. (2001). Heterogeneity of multiple sclerosis pathogenesis; implications for diagnosis and therapy. *Trends Mol Med,* 7:115-121.

Leary, S.M., Porter, B. & Thompson, A.J. (2005). Multiple sclerosis: diagnosis and the management of acute relapses. *Postgrad Med J,* 81:302-308.

Lublin, F.D. & Reingold, S.C. (1996). Defining the clinical course of multiple sclerosis: Results of an international survey. *Neurology,* 46:907-911.

Mameli, G., Astone, V., Arru, G., Marconi, S., Lovato, L., Serra, C., Sotgiu, S., Bonetti, B. & Dolei, A. (2007). Brains and peripheral blood mononuclear cells of multiple sclerosis (MS) patients hyper express MS-associated retrovirus/HERV-W endogenous retrovirus, but not Human herpes virus 6. *J Gen Virol,* 88:264-274.

Mancardi, G. & Saccardi, R. (2008). Autologous haematopoietic stem-cell transplantation in multiple sclerosis. *Lancet Neurol,* 7:626-636.

Mancuso, R., Delbue, S., Borghi, E., Pagani, E., Calvo, M.G., Caputo, D., Granieri, E. & Ferrante, P. (2007). Increased prevalence of varicella zoster virus DNA in cerebrospinal fluid from patients with multiple sclerosis. *J Med Virol,* 79:192-199.

Manzoli, F.A., Stefoni, S., Manzoli-Guidotti, L. & Barbieri, M. (1970). The fatty acids of myelin phospholipids. *FEBS Lett,* 10:317-320.

Martino, G. & Hartung, H.P. (1999). Immunopathogenesis of multiple sclerosis: the role of T-cells. *Curr Opin Neurol,* 12:309-321.

Matute, C. & Perez-Cerda, F. (2005). Multiple sclerosis: novel perspectives on newly forming lesions. *Trends Neurosci,* 28:173-175.

Matute, C., Alberdi, E., Domercq, M., Perez-Cerda, F., Perez-Samartin, A. & Sanchez-Gomez, M.V. 2001. The link between excitotoxic oligodendroglial death and demyelinating diseases. *Trends Neurosci,* 24:224-230.

Mayer, M. (1991). Linoleic acid – dependent slowing of erythrocyte sedimentation in multiple sclerosis. *Prostaglandins Leukot Essent Fatty Acids,* 44:257-258.

Miller, G. (2005). The dark side of glia. *Science,* 308:778-781.

Mitchell, D.C. & Litman, B.J. (2001). Modulation of receptor signaling by phospholipids acyl chain composition. In Mostofsky, D.I., Yehuda, S. & Salem, N. (eds). *Fatty acids. Physiological and behavioral functions*. Totowa, NJ: Humana Press: 23-40.

Modi, G., Mochan, A., Du Toit, M. & Stander, I. (2008). Multiple sclerosis in South Africa. *S Afr Med J,* 98:391-393.

Moses, H. Jr. & Sriram, S. 2001. An infectious basis for multiple sclerosis: perspectives on the role of Chlamydia pneumoniae and other agents. *BioDrugs,* 15:199-206.

Mouritsen, O.G. & Jørgensen, K. (1994). Dynamical order and disorder in lipid bilayers. *Chem Phys Lipids,* 73:3-25.

Mouritsen, O.G. & Jørgensen, K. (1998). A new look at lipid-membrane structure in relation to drug research. *Pharm Res,* 15:1507-1519.

Nakamura, M.T. & Nara, T.Y. (2004). Structure, function, and dietary regulation of Δ6, Δ5, and Δ9 desaturases. *Annu Rev Nutr,* 24:345-376.

Narasimhan, B., Mourya, V. & Dhake, A. (2006). Design, synthesis, antibacterial, and QSAR studies of myristic acid derivatives. *Bioorg Med Chem Lett,* 16:3023-3029.

Navarro, X. & Segura, R. (1989). Red blood cell fatty acids in multiple sclerosis. *Acta Neurol* Scand, 79:32-37.

Nielsen, T.R., Rostgaard, K., Nielsen, N.M., Koch-Hendriksen, N., Haahr, S., Sorensen, P.S. & Hjalgrim, H. (2007). Multiple sclerosis after infectious mononucleosis. *Arch Neurol,* 64:72-75.

Nightingale, S., Woo, E., Smith, A.D., French, J.M., Gale, M.M., Sinclair, H.M., Bates, D. & Shaw, D.A. (1990). Red blood cell and adipose tissue fatty acids in mild inactive multiple sclerosis. *Acta Neurol Scand,* 82:43-50.

Nordvik, I., Myhr, K.M., Nyland, H. & Bjerve, K.S. (2000). Effect of dietary advice and n-3 supplementation in newly diagnosed MS patients. *Acta Neurol Scand,* 102:143-149.

Noseworthy, J.H., Lucchinetti, C., Rodriguez, M. & Weinshenker, B.G. (2000). Multiple Sclerosis. *N Engl J Med,* 343:938-952.

Oka, A., Belliveau, M.J., Rosenberg, P.A. & Volpe, J.J. (1993). Vulnerability of oligodendroglia to glutamate: pharmacology, mechanisms, and prevention. *J Neurosci,* 13:1441-1453.

Okubo, K., Hamasaki, N., Hara, K. & Kageura, M. (1991). Palmitoylation of cysteine 69 from the COOH-terminal of Band 3 protein in the human erythrocyte membrane. *J Biol Chem,* 266:16420-16424.

Okuda, Y., Okuda, M., Apatoff, B.R. & Posnett, D.N. (2005). The activation of memory CD4+ T cells and CD8+ Tcells in patients with multiple sclerosis. *J Neurol Sci,* 235:11-17.

Paty, D.W., Cousin, H.K., Read, S. & Adlakha, K. (1978). Linoleic acid in multiple sclerosis: Failure to show any therapeutic benefit. *Acta Neurol Scand,* 58:53-58.

Pereira, S.L., Leonard, A.E. & Mukerji, P. (2003). Recent advances in the study of fatty acid desaturases from animals and lower eukaryotes. *Proataglandins Leukot Essent Fatty Acids,* 68: 97-106.

Perron, H., Lazarini, F., Ruprecht, K., Pechoux-Longin, C., Sellhean, D., Sazdovitch, V., Creange, A., Battall-Poirot, N., Sibal, G., Santoro, L. Jolivet, M., Darlix, J.L., Rieckmann, P., Arzberger, T., Hauw, J.J. & Lassmann, H. (2005). Human endogenous retrovirus (HERV)-W ENV and GAG proteins: physiological expression in human brain and pathophysiological modulation in multiple sclerosis lesions. *J Neurovirol,* 11:23-33.

Piani, D. & Fontana, A. (1994). Involvement of the cystine transport system xc- in the macrophage-induced glutamate-dependent cytotoxicity to neurons. *J Immunol,* 152:3578-3585.

Pino, A., Brescianini, S., D'Ippolito, C., Fagnani, C., Alimonti, A. & Stazi, M.A. (2005). *Discriminant analysis to study trace elements in biomonitoring: an application on neurodegenerative diseases.* Ann 1st Super Sanità, 41:223-228.

Pollock, S., Harrison, M.J. & O'Connell, G. (1982). Erythrocyte deformability in multiple sclerosis. *J Neurol Neurosurg Psychiatry,* 45:762.

Polman, C.H., Reingold, S.C., Edan, G., Filippi, M., Hartung, H-P., Kappos, L., Lublin, F.D., Metz, L.M., McFarland, H.F., O'Connor, P.W. Sandberg-Wollheim, M., Thompson, A.J., Weinshenker, B.G. & Wolinsky, J.S. (2005). Diagnostic criteria for multiple sclerosis: 2005 revisions to the "McDonald Criteria". *Ann Neurol,* 58:840-846.

Prineas, J.W. & Wright, R.G. (1978). Macrophages, lymphocytes, and plasma cells in the perivascular compartment in chronic multiple sclerosis. *Lab Invest,* 38:409-421.

Rapoport, S.I., Rao, J.S. & Igarashi, M. (2007). Brain metabolism of nutritionally essential polyunsaturated fatty acids depends on both the diet and the liver. *Prostaglandins Leukot Essent Fatty Acids,* 77:251-261.

Reipert, B. (2004). Multiple sclerosis: a short review of the disease and its differences between men and women. *The Journal of Men's Health & Gender,* 1:334-340.

Repovic, P., Kaihong, M.I. & Benveniste, E. N. (2003). Oncostatin M enhances the expression of prostaglandin E_2 and cyclooxygenase-2 in astrocytes: Synergy with interleukin-1β, tumor necrosis factor-α, and bacterial lipopolysaccharide. *Glia,* 42:433-446.

Roche, H.M. (1999). Unsaturated fatty acids. *Proc Nutr Soc,* 58:397-401.

Rola-Pleszezynski, M. & Stankova, J. (1992). Cytokine gene regulation by PGE2, LTB4 and PAF. *Mediat Inflamm,* 1:5-8

Romon, M., Nuttens, M.C., Theret, N., Delbart, C., Lecerf, J.M., Fruchart, J.C. & Salomez, J.L. (1995). Comparison between fat intake assessed by a 3-day food record and phospholipid fatty acid composition of red blood cells. *Metab Clin Exp,* 44:1139-1145.

Rosati, G. (2001). The prevalence of multiple sclerosis in the world: an update. *J Neurol Sci,* 22:117-139.

Sands, J.A. (1977). Inactivation and inhibition of replication of the enveloped bacteriophage φ6 by fatty acids. *Antimicrob Agents Chemother,* 12:523-528.

Schippling, S., Heesen, C., Zander, A. & Martin, R. (2008). Stem cell transplantation in multiple sclerosis. *J Neurol,* 255:43-47.

Sellner, J., Greeve, I. & Mattle, H.P. (2008). Atorvastatin decreases high-sensitivity C-reactive protein in multiple sclerosis. *Mult Scler,* 14:981-984.

Simopoulos, A.P. (2002). Omega-3 fatty acids in inflammation and autoimmune diseases. *J Am Coll Nutr,* 21:495-505.

Sotgiu, S., Arru, G., Mameli, G., Serra, C., Pugliatti, M., Rosati, G. & Dolei, A. (2006). Multiple sclerosis-associated retrovirus in early multiple sclerosis: a six-year follow-up of a Sardinian cohort. *Mult Scler,* 12:698-703.

Sprecher, H. (1982). Biochemistry of essential fatty acids. *Prog Lipid Res,* 20:13-22

Sprecher, H. (2000). Metabolism of highly unsaturated n-3 and n-6 fatty acids. *Biochim Biophys Acta,* 1486:219-231.

Stinissen, P., Raus, J. & Zhang J. (1997). Autoimmune pathogenesis of multiple sclerosis: role of autoreactive T lymphocytes and new immunotherapeutic strategies. *Crit Rev Immunol,* 17:33-75.

Tilley, S.L., Coffman, T.M. & Koller, B.H. (2001). Mixed messages: modulation of inflammation and immune responses by prostaglandins and thromboxanes. *J Clin Invest,* 108:15-23.

Toshniwal, P.K. & Zarling, E.J. (1992). Evidence for increased lipid peroxidation in multiple sclerosis. *Neurochem Res,* 17:205-207.

Tsang, W.M., Belin, J., Monro, J.A., Smith, A.D., Thompson, R.H.S. & Zilkha, K.J. (1976). Relationship between plasma and lymphocyte linoleate in multiple sclerosis. *J Neurol Neurosurg Psychiatry,* 39:767-71.

Van Meeteren, M.E., Teunissen, C.E., Dijkstra, C.D. & Van Tol, E.A.F. (2005). Antioxidants and polyunsaturated fatty acids in multiple sclerosis. *Eur J Clin Nutr,* 59:1347-1361.

Voet, D. & Voet, J.G. (1995). Lipids and membranes. In Rose, N. (ed). *Biochemistry.* 2nd ed. New York: John Wiley & Sons, Inc: 277-329.

Warren, S.A., Warren, K.G., Greenhill, S. & Paterson, M. (1982). How multiple sclerosis is related to animal illness, stress and diabetes. *Can Med Assoc J,* 126:377-385.

Weinstock-Guttman, B., Baier, M., Park, Y., Feichter, J., Lee-Kwen, P., Gallagher, E., Venkatraman, J., Meksawan, K., Deinehert, S., Pendergast, D., Awad, A.B., Ramanathan, M., Munschauer, F. & Rudick, R. (2005). Low fat dietary intervention with ω-3 fatty acid supplementation in multiple sclerosis patients. *Prostaglandins Leukot Essent Fatty Acids,* 73:397-404.

Westlund, K.B. & Kurland, L.T. (1953). Studies on multiple sclerosis in Winnipeg, Manitoba, and New Orleans, Louisiana. *Am J Hyg,* 57:397-407.

Willer, C.J. & Ebers, G.C. (2000). Susceptibility to multiple sclerosis: interplay between genes and environment. *Curr Opin Neurol,* 13:241-247.

Williams, E.E. (1998). Membrane lipids: What membrane physical properties are conserved during physiochemically-induced membrane restructuring? *Amer Zool,* 38:280-290.

Wilson, R. & Tocher, D.R. (1991). Lipid and fatty acid composition is altered in plaque tissue from multiple sclerosis brain compared with normal brain white matter. *Lipids,* 26:9-15.

Zamaria, N. (2004). Alteration of polyunsaturated fatty acid status and metabolism in health and disease. *Reprod Nutr Dev,* 44:273-282.

Zeis, T., Graumann, U., Reynolds, R. & Schaeren-Wiemers, N. (2008). Normal-appearing white matter in multiple sclerosis is in a subtle balance between inflammation and neuroprotection. *Brain,* 131:288-303.

Zhang, S.M., Willett, W.C., Hernán, M.A., Olek, M.J. & Ascherio, A. (2000). Dietary fat in relation to risk of multiple sclerosis among two large cohorts of women. *Am J Epidemiol,* 152:1056-1064.

In: Multiple Sclerosis
Editor: E. Scholz and C. Müller, pp. 59-79

ISBN 978-1-61324-848-5

Chapter III

Multiple Sclerosis: Causes, Diagnosis and Management

Georgia Deretzi, Emmanuel Gavalas, Christos Zavos, Stergios A. Polyzos, Dimitrios Tsiptsios, Evangelia Giartza-Taxidou, Iakovos Tsiptsios and Jannis Kountouras*

Department of Medicine, Second Medical Clinic, Aristotle University of Thessaloniki, Hippokration Hospital, Thessaloniki, Greece

Abstract

Multiple sclerosis (MS) is an organ-specific inflammatory demyelinating disease of the central nervous system (CNS) mediated by autoreactive T lymphocytes with specificity for myelin self-antigens; it affects more than two million people worldwide and has been recognized as the leading cause of neurological disability among young adults.

MS is a multi-factorial and multigenic disorder, in which an infectious agent on a genetically permissive host can result in inflammation, demyelination and neuro-degeneration. The major genetic factor in MS is the major histocompatibility complex (MHC), affecting both the immune repertoire and regulatory circuits, and the DRB*1501 allele; other susceptibility genes such as interleukin (IL)-7 and IL-2 receptors have been additionally identified. Among environmental factors such as decreased vitamin D, stress and smoking, infections are emerging as the most consistent predictors of MS risk; genes and infections by pathogens might act synergistically to trigger the disease. In this respect, the possibility that microorganisms can cause MS has recently been addressed; Epstein-Barr virus, human herpes virus-6, *Chlamydia pneumoniae*, and possibly *Helicobacter pylori* (*Hp*) may cause the neurological damage that results in MS.

Neuroinflammation might initiate from the periphery and relative data suggest that activated encephalitogenic immune effectors [T helper cell (Th)1, Th17, CD8 cells, B

* Correspondence to: Jannis Kountouras, MD, PhD, Professor of Medicine, Gastroenterologist, 8 Fanariou St, Byzantio, 551 33, Thessaloniki, Macedonia, Greece. Tel: +30-2310-892238, Fax: +30-2310-992794; E-mail: jannis@auth.gr.

cells, and macrophages], through the disrupted blood-brain barrier, powerfully influence the processes in the brain. Active inflammation, marked by augmented numbers of activated and primed microglia, increased steady-state levels of inflammatory cytokines and decreases in anti-inflammatory molecules, may determine the initial phase of the disease. In the CNS, an immunological cascade, consisting of epitope spreading, triggers the activation of the innate immune system (microglia, dendritic cells, astrocytes, B cells), which leads to chronic inflammation. Demyelination is observed in both white and gray matter of the CNS. Four different pathological patterns (Lassmann's patterns) have been identified in the lesions in the brain tissue (pattern I: T-cell-mediated; pattern II: T-cell plus antibody-mediated autoimmune response; patterns III and IV: highly suggestive of a primary oligodendrocyte dystrophy).

Several clinical forms of MS have been described such as relapsing-remitting MS (RRMS), secondary progressive, primary progressive and progressive-relapsing. This classification is important both for prognosis and therapeutic decisions. RRMS is characterized by unpredictable relapses followed by periods of remission. Approximately 10% of patients begin with a primary progressive form of the disease being the most disabling.

MS symptoms develop as the cumulative result of multiple lesions in the brain and spinal cord. Neurological symptoms include visual problems, changes in sensation, muscle weakness, ataxia, fatigue, bladder and bowel difficulties, cognitive impairment and emotional symptoms.

Diagnosis is based on the McDonald criteria focusing on clinical, laboratory and radiologic data of the dissemination MS lesions in time and space. The most commonly used diagnostic tools are magnetic resonance imaging, analysis of the cerebrospinal fluid for oligoclonal bands of immunoglobulin G and evoked potential.

Although the cure of MS is unknown, a multidisciplinary approach has proven to be helpful. Management aims to restore the function after a relapse (using intravenous administration of high doses of corticosteroids) and to prevent new relapses and disability (using disease-modifying treatments or immunosuppressors). MS medications and rehabilitation programs (physiotherapy, neurocognitive and psychological rehabilitation) improve the quality of life of MS patients. Expectedly, *Hp* eradication might alter the initiation and/or progression of MS.

Introduction

Multiple sclerosis (MS) is a common and severe central nervous system (CNS) disorder characterized by myelin loss, chronic inflammation, axonal and oligodendrocyte pathology, and progressive neurological dysfunction. Extensive epidemiological data confirm that genetic variation is an essential determinant of susceptibility to MS and suggest that such variation also influences the timing of symptom onset, the course of the disease and the treatment response. MS is considered to be a chronic T cell-mediated autoimmune disease that results in the presence of inflammation, demyelination and neurodegeneration within the CNS. Worldwide, the incidence of MS is approximately 0.1%; it has been recognized as the leading cause of neurological disability among young adults with substantial impact in social life, cost of healthcare and loss of wages. The average age of onset is between 20 and 40. It is rare in children and after the age of 65 years. The age is an important factor related to the course and prognosis of MS. MS is most prevalent among Caucasians particularly those of European ancestry, with a female-to-male ratio of approximately 2:1; women are more susceptible to MS than men and accumulating evidence indicates that the incidence and prevalence of MS is increasing more so in women than in men [1].

Etiology

The etiology of MS is an elusive field due to the lack of the standard cause–effect relationship model to explain the disease. Despite the enormous hard work made in MS research, the pathogenic mechanisms involved in the inflammatory and degenerative process of MS are still unclear.

Accumulating evidence indicates that MS is an organ-specific autoimmune disease mediated by autoreactive T lymphocytes (TLs) with specificity for myelin self-antigens [2]. A breakdown of central and peripheral tolerance leads to the survival and eventual activation of aberrant autoreactive TLs, key contributors to the underlying pathogenetic mechanisms responsible for onset and progression of MS [3]. Furthermore other immune components such as T regulatory cells (Tregs), T helper cell (Th)17, B cells and other components of the innate immune system act synergistically in MS pathogenesis [2,3]. The female predominance of MS [4], the tendency for remission of the disease during pregnancy [5], the evidence from experimental autoimmune encephalomyelitis [6], the response to immunomodulatory therapy [7], and the coexistence of MS with other autoimmune diseases [8] further support the concept that MS shares many clinical and pathological characteristics of autoimmune diseases.

Current data suggest that MS is a heterogeneous multi-factorial and multi-genic disease, where an infective agent on a genetically permissive host can result in neurological damage of CNS accompanied by dysregulation of immune system. Multiple infectious agents including herpes viruses, coronaviruses, retroviruses and synchronous infections have been implicated in the pathogenesis of MS with variable findings depending on the agent, techniques and disease phenotype. Inflammatory brain lesions appear to arise from autoimmune responses involving activated lymphocytes and monocytes. Major histocompatibility complex (MHC) is the consistent susceptibility locus in MS. Polymorphisms in DR gene (the *HLA-DR15* haplotype on chromosome 6p21.3, DRB*1501 allele) is the primary contributor to MS susceptibility, affecting both the immune repertoire and regulatory circuits. Moreover, recent findings in non-HLA genes as well as their single nucleotide polymorphisms SNPs have shown high linkage to MS as a genetic-based disorder; single nucleotide polymorphisms in the α chain of the interleukin-7 (IL-7) and IL-2 receptors and novel MS susceptibility loci such as IL-22RA2 have been additionally identified [9,10]. Although genetic susceptibility explains the familial clustering of MS and the sharp decline in risk with increasing genetic distance, it cannot completely explain the geographical variations in the MS frequency and the changes in risk that occur with migration, which strongly support the implication of environmental factors (Figure 1).

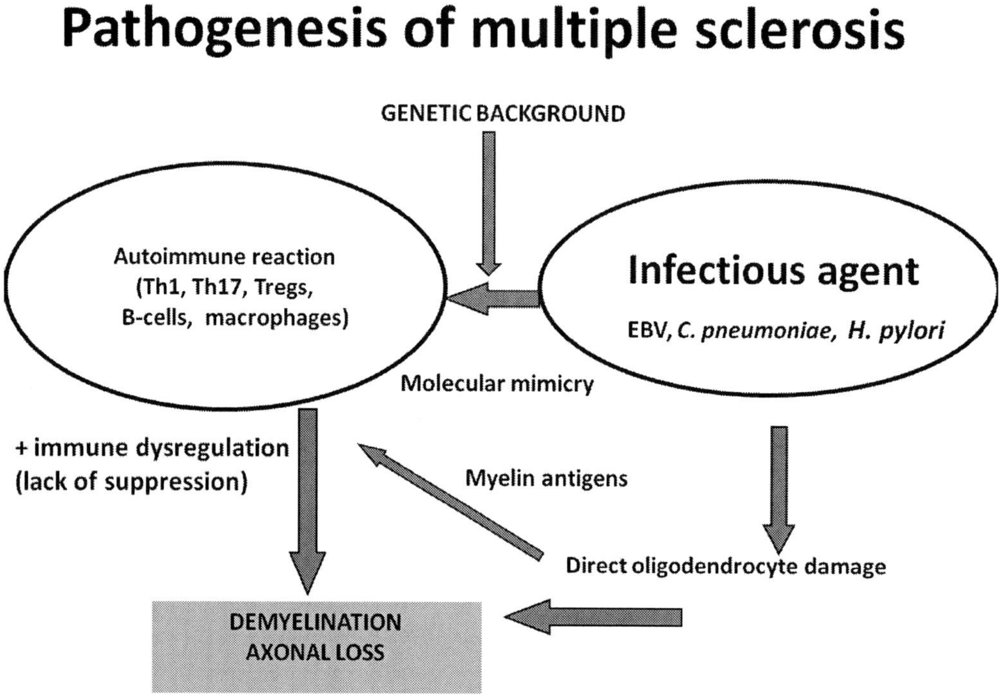

Figure 1. Interaction between susceptibility genes and environmental factors (i.e., infectious agents) is an important player in the pathogenesis of multiple sclerosis. An infectious agent on a genetically permissive host acts synergistically with dysregulation of immune system or/and directly damage oligodendrocytes, resulting in inflammation, demyelination and axonal loss in the CNS. (Th, T helper cells; EBV, Epstein-Barr virus; *C. pneumoniae*, *Chlamydia pneumoniae*; *H. pylori*, *Helicobacter pylori*)

Immunopathophysiology

Phase 1: Initial Phase, Systemic Infections

The evidence that the environment acts long before MS becomes clinically evident is well established and suggests the existence of a prodromal phase for the disease. Among environmental factors such as decreased sunlight, vitamin D, stress, diet and smoking, infections are emerging as the most consistent predictors of MS risk; the interplay between susceptibility genes and environmental factors is considered an important player in the genesis of MS and a role for an infectious pathogen has long been considered central to the disease process. In this regard, genes and infections by pathogens might act synergistically to trigger the disease [11,12].

A growing body of evidence suggests that systemic infections are a risk factor for the initiation of autoimmune processes including the induction of acute events in MS; although the early events in MS remain uncertain, active systemic inflammation may determine the initial phase of the disease. Importantly, inappropriate in time, place and extent inflammation is progressively incriminated in diverse disease conditions including, most relevant here, CNS pathologies. The persistence of oligoclonal bands of immunoglobulin G (IgG) is consistent with infectious or parainfectious disorders of the CNS. Neuroinflammation might initiate from the periphery and relative data suggest that peripheral conditions, through the disrupted blood-brain barrier (BBB), powerfully influence various pathologic processes in the brain including MS [13]; infections by pathogens such as Epstein-Barr virus, human herpes virus (HSV) 6, *Chlamydia pneumoniae (C. pneumoniae*) and *Helicobacter pylori* (*Hp*) might act synergistically with genes to induce or trigger MS [12,14-16]. Infection-induced molecular mimicry can trigger MS by eliciting inflammation which may cause the neurological damage that results in MS [17]. Notably, the communicable factor is acquired in early adolescence [18].

Phase 2: Invasion of Activated Encephalitogenic Immune Effectors into the CNS

The activated encephalitogenic immune effectors (Th1, Th17, CD8+ cells, B cells, and macrophages) from the periphery express surface molecules that allow them to penetrate the BBB and enter the CNS [19]. However, the explanation of the initial process of breakdown of normally tight BBB and the association of cellular infiltration into the CNS remains unanswered. In this regard, a series of factors have been implicated in BBB disruption including inflammatory mediators [e.g., cytokines and chemokines induced by *Hp* infection (*Hp*-I)] and oxidative stress [20,21]. Specifically, current *Hp*-I induces humoral and cellular immune responses that, owing to the sharing of homologous epitopes (molecular mimicry), cross-react with host components, thereby contributing and possibly perpetuating neural tissue damage [22]. Moreover, eradicating *Hp*-I may alter MS pathophysiology. *Hp* could indirectly affect the brain and other target organs through the release of numerous cytokines such as tumor necrosis factor (TNF)-α acting at a distance; TNF-α is involved in BBB disruption through a mechanism involving matrix metalloproteinases upregulation [23]. In addition, *Hp*-induced cytotoxin VacA exhibits chemotactic activities to the bone marrow-derived mast cells (BMDMCs) and induces BMDMCs to produce proinflammatory cytokines including TNF-α; BMDMCs reside adjacent to blood and lymphatic channels, mainly under epithelial surfaces including the BBB and gastrointestinal tract [24,25]. *Hp* stimulates mast cells directly or via gastrin induction and mast cells are actively involved in the pathogenesis of *Hp*-associated pathologies [23]. Apart from activated mast cells, vascular endothelial growth factor (VEGF), IL-8, chymase or tryptase (a serine endoprotease released by mast cells) and mast cell growth factor linked to *Hp*-I, mast cells themselves can be stimulated by corticotropin-releasing hormone, secreted under stress, to release mediators including histamine, IL-8, tryptase and VEGF, which disrupt the BBB [23,26,27]. In turn, BBB breakdown could promote entry of immune cells (autoreactive effector CD4+ and CD8+ T cells) infiltrations, activated monocytes infected with *Hp,* due to defective autophagy resulting in *Hp* replication in autophagic vesicles [28] and/or *Hp* circulating antibodies into the central neurons resulting in the development of neuronal pathologies, possibly including MS. In this regard, apart from pathogens' intranasal inoculation, the influx of activated monocytes infected with *C. pneumoniae* through the BBB could have dire consequences in the brain leading to the development of degenerative diseases, including MS.

Phase 3: Inflammation - Demyelination

Inflammation, demyelination, axonal and neuronal damage within the CNS are recognized to be the pathological features of MS and the critical components in the progression of the disease (Table 1).

Table 1. Immunopathogenesis of multiple sclerosis (MS)

Evidence of inflammation/demyelination	Evidence of degeneration
• Accumulation of autoreactive CD4+ T cells B cells and plasma cells in MS lesions • Invasion of CD8+ T cells, γδ T cells and macrophages in parenchyma. • Ectopic meningeal B-cell follicles. • Activation of Th1 and Th17 pro-inflammatory responses; production of TNF-α, TNF-β, IFN-γ, IL-12, IL-2, IL-17 • Production of chemokines, lymphotoxin, matrix metalloproteinases • Presence of oligoclonal bands in CSF • Antibodies production • Coexistence with other autoimmune diseases • Inflammatory lesions in MRI (Gd+) • Response to immunotherapies • Acute EAE model	• Activated astrocytes and microglia • Production of reactive species, excitotoxicity, autoantibody production • Axonal loss is independent to inflammation • Oligodendrocytes apoptosis • Accumulation of APP in active lesions • Axonal transection/degeneration in active lesions • Reduction in axonal density in normal appearing white matter in MS • Oxidative damage in mitochondrial DNA • Impaired activity of mitochondrial enzyme complexes • Complement mediated cytotoxicity • Nitric oxide mediates to axonal damage • CNS atrophy and T1 hypointense lesion load in MRI • NAA reduction and magnetization transfer ratios of normal appearing brain matter • Chronic EAE model; CD8+ lymphocytes

Evidence of inflammation, demyelination and degeneration are hallmarks in the pathogenesis of MS. (EAE, experimental autoimmune encephalomyelitis; CSF, cerebrospinal fluid; TNF, tumor-necrosis factor; IFN-γ, interferon-γ; IL, interleukin; MRI, magnetic resonance imaging; NAA, *N*-acetyl-aspartate; APP, amyloid precursor protein)

Demyelinated plaques are distributed throughout the CNS around a medium size vessel. The demyelinating process is associated with persistent inflammation; inflammation is not restricted to the areas of demyelination but also affects the normal-appearing white and grey matter, and, to a lesser extent, the meninges [29,30].

Activated immune effectors (T-, B- cells and macrophages), through the disrupted BBB, powerfully influence the processes in the brain. Active plaques occur early during the disease and are characterized by the presence of mononuclear cells including T-, B- cells and macrophages in brain perivascular spaces. In the CNS, an immunological cascade consisting of epitope spreading, triggers the activation of the innate immune system (microglia, dendritic cells, astrocytes, B cells), which leads to chronic inflammation. Active inflammation, marked by augmented numbers of activated and primed microglia, increased steady-state levels of inflammatory cytokines and decreases in anti-inflammatory molecules, may determine the initial phase of the disease [29-31]. Notably, the 'cross-talk' between mast cells, lymphocytes, neurons and glia constitutes a neuroimmune axis implicated in a range of neurodegenerative diseases with an inflammatory and/or autoimmune component.

Both the innate and the ill-fated adaptive immune responses can potentially contribute to the etiopathogenesis of MS. In the recent years the contribution of innate immune cells in mediating MS pathogenesis is being evaluated; anti-inflammatory or pro-inflammatory function of dendritic cells, microglial cells, natural killer (NK) cells, NK-T cells and γδ T cells, along with their interaction among themselves and with myelin, contribute to MS pathophysiology. Moreover, the discovery of Th17 cells but also IL-17-secreting γδ T cells and their association with neuroinflammation has broken the dogma that interferon (IFN)-γ-producing Th1 cells have the exclusive capacity to invade and destroy the CNS tissue. In this regard, during active MS disease, inflammatory Th1/Th17 cells predominate over immunoregulatory Th2/Treg cells; CD4+CD25+ Tregs play a key role in the control of self-antigen-reactive T cells and the maintenance of peripheral tolerance, which may be diminished in MS. Forkhead box p3 (FOXp3), a transcriptional factor, has been identified as the molecular programmer of Tregs focused on suppressive function [32,33].

Specifically, MS is crucially dependent on the activation of pro-inflammatory Th1 T cells by antigen-presenting cells, resistance of T cells to Fas-mediated apoptosis is involved in its exacerbation and auto-aggressive Th1 cells can be adoptively transferred to non-diseased recipient mice that subsequently develop the disease [34]. MHC class II restricted TLs polarized to the production of inflammatory Th1-type cytokines (IL-12, INF-γ and TNF-α); the interaction of activated CD4+ T cells with microglia and neurons led to a pro-inflammatory Th1 response with a Th1-type cytokine expression profile involved in the pathogenesis of apoptotic neuronal cell death in MS [36]. Activated T cells also produce TNF–β which generates apoptosis in oligodendrocytes in cultures. Notably, apoptotic rather than necrotic microglia-associated neurons' death appears as likely to underlie a number of common neurological conditions including MS [36]. Although CD4+ T cells are traditionally considered the main actors in MS immunopathology, multiple lines of evidence suggest that CD8+ T cells are also implicated in the pathogenesis; the CD8+ T cells detected in MS lesions demonstrate characteristics of activated and clonally expanded cells, thereby supporting the concept that these cells actively contribute to the observed injury.

Macrophages and activated microglia also participate in the induction of tissue damage in the acute plaques. As part of the inflammatory process, toxic macrophage products such as proteases, free radicals, nitric acid and perforins, cause myelin and oligodendrocytes' damage [37]; reactive oxygen species leading to oxidative stress, generated in excess primarily by macrophages, have been implicated as mediators of demyelination and axonal damage in MS.

B cells through their products immunoglobulins, their antigen-presenting and regulatory functions and cytokine secreting role have been also implicated in immune responses and in the degeneration of the axons in the inflammatory process of MS; there is an increasing body of evidence for the involvement of B cells and autoantibodies in the pathology of this disease, providing a rationale for treatments directed against B cells. An additional component involved in the progression of MS may be the presence of ectopic meningeal B-cell follicles. Activated B cells present in these structures produce chemokines that further attract other immune effectors [38,39].

Four different pathological patterns (Lassmann's patterns) have been identified in the plaques of the brain tissue (pattern I: T-cell-mediated; pattern II: T-cell plus antibody-mediated autoimmune response; patterns III and IV: highly suggestive of an oligodendrocyte dystrophy) providing information about differences in disease type and prognosis, and perhaps with different responses to treatment [30]. Patterns III and IV were highly supported by Prineas suggesting that the primary visible event appears to be the apoptotic death of oligodendrocytes [40].

Neurodegeneration begins early, even before progression appears clinically. Although axonal damage is more prominent in active inflammatory lesions, independent axonal and neuronal loss can be observed early on in MS, not only within active focal lesions but also in chronic silent plaques and in normal-appearing white and grey matter, as demonstrated pathologically [41] (Table 1). Axonal loss and neurofilament phosphorylation changes accompany lesion development and clinical progression in MS [42]. Of note, MS is active even during remission periods [43]. The chronic plaques are characterized by minimal inflammation and a broad astrocytic proliferation.

Apart from the usually known white matter demyelination, the cortex and deep gray matter are affected together with diffuse injury of the normal-appearing white matter [29,30]. Gray matter atrophy is independent of the MS lesions and is associated with physical disability, fatigue and cognitive impairment in MS [44].

Diagnosis

MS is usually considered a 'young persons' disease', characteristically presenting between the ages of 20 and 40. However, a relapsing pattern of the disease is not infrequent even in patients diagnosed over the age of 60. Active inflammation (clinical relapses and gadolinium enhancement) occurs in a significant number of patients with MS with later diagnosis, thereby having implications for the evaluation and treatment of patients with MS presenting at an older age.

In clinical practice, the process of diagnosis of MS may include:

- disease classification
- diagnosis confirmation, based on definite criteria
- alternative diagnosis exclusion

I. Clinical Classification

Subtypes or forms of MS have been described according to frequency and severity of neurological symptoms, the ability of the CNS to recover and the progression of the disease. Clinical forms widely used are relapsing-remitting multiple sclerosis (RRMS), secondary progressive (SPMS), primary progressive (PPMS) and progressive-relapsing (PRMS) (Figure 2). This classification is important both for the prognosis and for therapeutic decisions or response to specific treatments; it does not reflect pathologically different types of the disease [1,45,46].

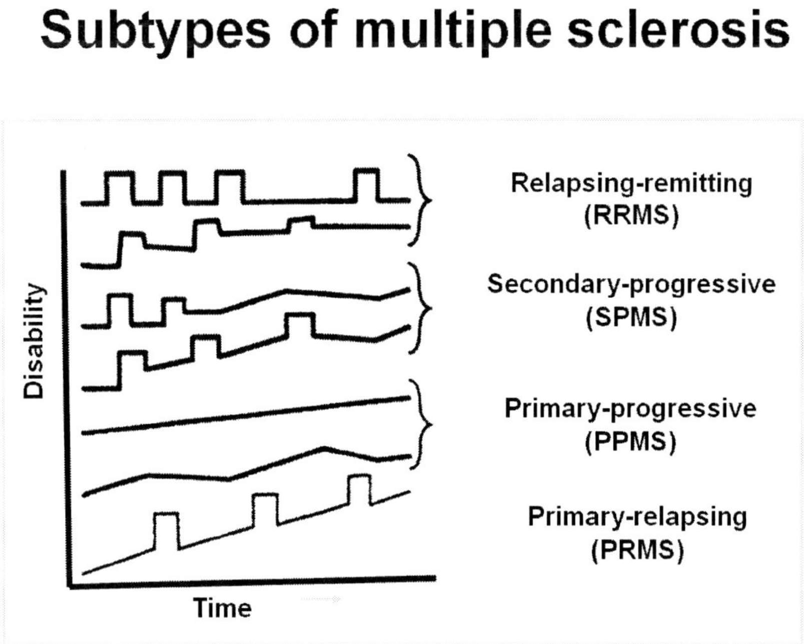

Figure 2. Clinical subtypes of multiple sclerosis: relapsing-remitting multiple sclerosis (RRMS), secondary progressive (SPMS), primary progressive (PPMS) and progressive-relapsing (PRMS). Classification is based on the appearance of relapses and remissions or/and progression of disability from the onset with or without remission.

The RRMS represents the initial course of approximately 85% of individuals with MS; it is characterized by unpredictable attacks (relapses or exacerbations) followed by remission (periods of months to years of relative clinically inactive disease). Deficits during attacks may either completely resolve or leave deficits. The RRMS usually begins with an attack suggestive of demyelinating disease but does not fulfill the criteria for MS. This is called clinically isolated syndrome (CIS); 30 to 70% of persons with a CIS later develop MS [47].

SPMS initiates as relapsing-remmiting form, which later (after a median time of 19 years) appears with a progressive deterioration of neurologic function, without remission. About 50% of people with RRMS develop SPMS during the first 10 years [48].

The PPMS represents approximately 10% of MS; it is characterized by progression of disability from the onset without remission. The age of onset for the PPMS subtype is around 40 years of age. PPMS patients develop ambulatory disability 50% faster than patients with RRMS.

Less common MS subtypes include PRMS, benign and malignant MS. In PRMS from the onset there is a steady neurologic decline with clear attacks. Benign MS was defined as subtype with low disability score (Expanded Disability Status Scale (EDSS) $\leq$3.0) at least 10 years after disease onset [49]. The malignant MS has a rapid progressive course leading to a significant disability with multiple neurological symptoms or death in a relatively short time after disease onset.

MS also behaves differently in childhood (pediatric form). MS pediatric form has more posterior fossa location, it takes more time to reach the progressive stage and may be distinguished from acute disseminated encephalomyelitis (ADEM) [50]; due to the confusing differential diagnosis of MS in children with other demyelinating diseases such as ADEM, it is important to reach this diagnosis when there is proof of white matter lesions disseminated in time and space that cannot be explained by any other mechanisms or pathologies. Late onset MS in aging is often primary progressive and polysymptomatic [51].

Balo concentric sclerosis, Schilder's diffuse sclerosis and Marburg disease are atypical variants of MS; whether they are MS variants or different diseases is controversial [52].

II. Confirmation of the Diagnosis Based on Definite Criteria

IIa. Clinical Criteria

History, clinical picture and physical examination serve as the basis for the diagnosis of MS in association with laboratory and imaging studies. Initial MS symptoms are monofocal or multifocal and develop as the cumulative result of multiple lesions in the brain and spinal cord. Diffuse symptoms such as dementia, behavior changes or loss of consciousness are rare. Most common presenting neurological symptoms of MS include muscle weakness, changes in sensation (hypoesthesia and paresthesia), visual problems (optic neuritis, diplopia, nystagmus), ataxia (deficit of coordination and balance), fatigue, bladder or bowel difficulties and cognitive impairment. The three most common CIS symptoms suggesting MS include those affecting the optic nerve, brain stem and spinal cord [1].

Objective documentation of neurological dissemination in time and space remain fundamental key of the diagnosis. Although the only proven diagnosis of MS is autopsy, non-invasive MS diagnosis is based on the McDonald criteria focusing on clinical, laboratory and radiologic data of the dissemination of MS lesions in time and space [47,53,54].

The main clinically used scale of disability progression and symptom severity is the EDSS [55]. Lhermitte's sign, an electrical sensation that runs down the spinal cord when bending the neck, is characteristic symptom of MS, though not specific [1,45].

IIb. Paraclinical Diagnostic Tools

In patients with symptoms and clinical examination indicating MS the most commonly used paraclinical diagnostic tools are magnetic resonance imaging (MRI) of the brain and spinal cord, analysis of the crebrospinal fluid (CSF) for oligoclonal bands and evoked potentials (EPs).

IIb1. Neuroimaging

MRI is a useful tool for MS diagnosis, the study of MS pathology and a marker of treatment efficacy and response; it is the best paraclinical tool currently available. Conventional MRI shows characteristic lesions of demyelination, existence of old lesions (not associated with symptoms at the moment of the evaluation), atrophy of the cortex and active plaques (highlighted by gadolinium enhancement). High-field MRI and more specific MR advanced techniques (proton MR spectroscopy, magnetization transfer imaging, diffusion tensor imaging) provide insights into the pathogenesis of MS and the impact of neuroprotective therapies. As surrogate markers of neurodegeneration, cortical atrophy, T1 hypointense lesion load, *N*-acetyl-aspartate levels or magnetization transfer ratios of normal-appearing brain matter have been used [47, 56, 57]. The MRI findings are unspecific for MS and may be differentiated from other alternative conditions with similar MRI appearance (mimicking MS lesions). For instance, in young patients with migraine or vasculitis and patients older than 50 years with cerebrovascular disorders with recurrent neurological symptoms, MRI findings that closely resemble those of MS may appear.

IIb2. CSF

CSF from a patient with MS analyzed by electrophoresis often shows a split to form so-called oligoclonal bands (OCBs). OCBs consist of proteins from activated lymphocytes and plasma cell clones; they are the most useful and accurate test for MS; it is an inflammation marker found in 85 to 90% of MS patients and should be compared with serum samples to rule out other diagnoses [58]. Furthermore, elevated IgG intrathecal synthesis rate and IgG index are inflammation markers in CSF. Apart from the above-mentioned immunological changes, the CSF is regularly normal in MS.

IIb3. EPs

EPs [visual (VEPs), brainstem auditory (BAEPs) and short latency somatosensory upper (USSEPs) and lower (LSSEPs)] are mainly useful when physical and neuroimaging findings do not establish the diagnosis of MS. In 75% of MS patients EPs are abnormal. EPs abnormalities do not justify conclusions about their utility value in diagnosis of MS, since they are present in a broad variety of CNS diseases.

Summarizing the aforementioned diagnostic methods, the sensitivity of MRI criteria is between 35 and 100%, and the specificity is between 36 and 92%. CSF oligoclonal banding shows sensitivities between 69 and 91% and specificities between 59 and 94%. Combination studies of MRI and CSF indicate enhanced sensitivity (56-100%) and specificity (53-96%) [59,60]. Studies on EPs did not justify conclusions about their value. A combination of clinical symptoms and simplified MRI criteria with CSF may be the best approach for an early MS diagnosis [61]. However, the value of a very early diagnosis stays questionable as the patients' benefit from the new diagnostic criteria has certainly not been addressed.

III. Differential Diagnosis

Differential diagnosis mainly includes systemic disorders (infectious, neoplastic, congenital, metabolic or vascular diseases) and non-MS idiopathic inflammatory demyelinating diseases of the CNS. Systemic disorders such as systemic lupus erythematosus, Sjögren's syndrome, sarcoidosis, CNS vasculitis, antiphospholipid syndrome, Lyme's disease involving the CNS and mimicking MS must be excluded [59,62]. Specifically, idiopathic inflammatory demyelinating diseases such as ADEM, neuromyelitis optica (NMO) and opticospinal MS in Asian population are conditions different from MS in course, pathophysiology, treatment, and prognosis. For instance, the discovery of NMO-IgG helps the clinicians to distinguish NMO from MS [63,64] (Table 2).

Table 2. Differential diagnosis of multiple sclerosis

Congenital disorders	adrenaleukodystrophy CADASIL Fabry disease metachromatic leukodystrophy mitochodrial disorders
Hematological manifestations	hemolytic anemia thrombotic thrombocytopenic purpura
Connective tissue disorders	antiphospholipid antibody syndrome Behçet disease systemic lupus erythematosus Sjögren's syndrome sarcoidosis
Cerebrovascular disorders	CADASIL hypertensive ischemic disease hypoxic-ischemic conditions lacunar infarcts Susac syndrome primary CNS vasculitis
Viral infections affective the CNS	
Malignancies	glioma lymphoma metastases paraneoplastic syndromes
Deficiency disorders	vitamin B12 deficiency Wilson's disease
Gastroenterological disorders	hepatic encephalopathy Whipple's disease
HIV-related diseases	progressive multifocal leukoencelophathy (JC virus)
Idiopathic inflammatory demyelinating diseases	acute disseminated encephalomyelitis (ADEM) neuromyelitis optica (NMO)

Natural History of MS

The course of MS results from the interplay of two clinical processes, relapses and progression. The disease appears on average at the age of 30 and follows a remitting or a progressive course in 85% and 15% of the cases, respectively. Early symptoms are related to an isolated or combined disturbance(s) of the long tracts of the CNS, the brainstem or the optic nerve in 70%, 20% and 25% of the cases, respectively. The relapse rate is one relapse on average every other year. After an exacerbating-remitting onset of MS, secondary progression occurs after 19 years on average. The median time to reach the landmarks of irreversible disability is 8 years regarding limitation of ambulation, 20 years for walking with a stick and 30 years for wheel-chair dependency. Characteristics of relapses early in the disease and the occurrence of a progressive phase seem to be the most reliable prognostic factors. Recent data suggest that the progressive phase in MS could be an age-dependent degenerative process, independent of previous relapses, and that the initial course of the disease does not substantially influence age at disability milestones. By contrast, a younger age at disease onset strongly correlates with a younger age when reaching disability landmarks, confirming that even if it takes longer for younger patients to accumulate irreversible disability, they are disabled at a younger age than patients with a later onset; patients with childhood onset reach these different critical phases of the disease at a younger age than patients with adult onset, thereby contradicting the notion of a more favorable prognosis in this age group [1,48,49].

Management

Although the cure of MS is unknown, a multidisciplinary approach has proven to be helpful. Paradoxically, during the last two decades a plethora of therapeutics were brought to the market for MS treatment. The heterogeneity of MS (diversity of MS lesions/MS subtypes), the uncertainty of the natural history and treatment efficacy in individual MS patients in addition to the absence of identification of reliable biological surrogate markers, frequently pose a dilemma to the clinician. The efficacy of therapy is rather limited, due to inadequate and non-specific eradication of autoimmune cells; irreversible damage (axonal loss, atrophy); and side effects appearance. Nevertheless, the defective remyelinating/ regenerating mechanisms could account for this. The annualized relapses rate, MRI lesions changes and progression of disability might be considered as parameters for therapeutic efficacy. Of note, management of symptoms in MS has received little attention compared with disease-modifying treatments. However, the effect of these symptoms on the quality of life can be profound.

Current management for MS includes:

- Treatment of relapses
- Modification of the course of the disease
- Symptomatic medications
- Rehabilitation programs
- Treatment of Relapses

A relapse due to an episode of acute inflammation within the CNS is a neurological event that lasts more than 24 hours and is independent of heat exposure, infection or fever. MS temporal relapses are often unpredictable, occurring without caution or obvious provocative factors. Some attacks, however, are preceded by common triggers such as stress or infections, and are more frequent in the first few months after delivery. The decision to treat relapses depends on the increase in disability and the functional impact on daily activities. Acute severe episodes (including optic neuritis or traverse myelitis) should be treated by a course of high-dose corticosteroids started immediately after the onset of the relapse with intravenous methylprednisolone (500–1000 mg daily for three or five days). Intravenous immunoglobulin

(IG, IVIG 0.4 g/kg/d for 5 days) and plasma exchange may be alternative option of severe relapses in pregnant women, in patients refractory to steroids or in whom steroid use is contraindicated [65,66].

Modification of the Course of the Disease

Theoretically, MS should be controlled by blocking or reversing the immunological mechanisms involved in the pathogenesis of the disease. Targeting these mechanisms in general, may be efficacious in preventing MS (Figure 3). For instance, natalizumab and FTY720 target leukocyte trafficking and antigen-specific therapies binding on the antigen-specific T-cell receptor (TCR) to peptide/MHC class II complexes on the surface of antigen-presenting cells triggers the initial activation of T cells.

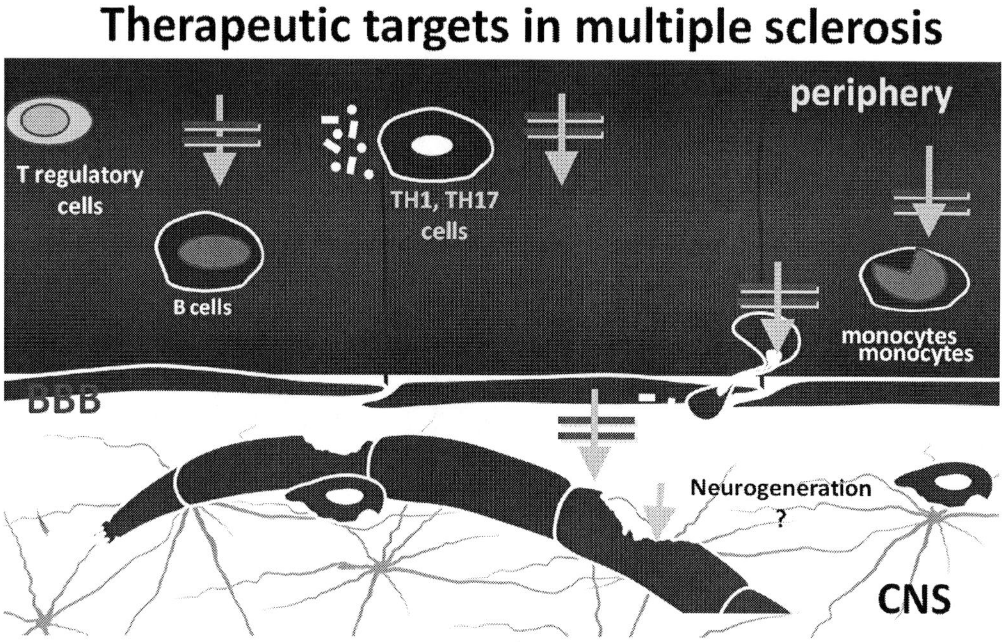

Figure 3. Therapeutic targets in multiple sclerosis (MS) based on the pathogenesis. MS should be controlled by blocking or reversing the immunological mechanisms at different levels involved in the pathogenesis of the disease. Blockade of activated immune effectors [T helper (Th)1 cells, Th17 cells, CD8+ cells, B cells and macrophages] from the periphery to penetrate the blood–brain barrier and enter the central nervous system (CNS); preservation of peripheral tolerance by innate immune system and endorsement of regulatory T cell and anti-inflammatory Th2 are potential therapeutic targets. In the CNS, autoreactive immune effectors together with abnormally-activated microglia and astrocytes cause inflammation, demyelination and axonal loss. Neuroprotection and prevention of neurodegeneration are still under investigation (BBB, blood-brain barrier).

Goals in the therapy of MS focus on reducing symptoms and disease progression. Therefore, long-term follow-up studies are needed to elucidate the impact of disease-modifying therapies (DMTs) in MS [67]. Immunomodulation is preferable to immuno-suppression since it targets the relevant autoimmune cells specifically or, alternatively, it enhances the existing suppressive/control mechanisms of the immune system.

During the last twenty years five DMTs, widely used for RRMS modifying the course of the disease, have been able to reduce MRI activity and frequency of exacerbations approximately by 30%. First-line DMTs for MS approved by regulatory agencies include the following medications: IFN-β-1b (Betaseron and Extavia, subcutaneous injection, every other day), IFN-β-1a (Avonex, intramuscular injection once per week, and Rebif, subcutaneous injection three times per week), and glatiramer acetate (Copaxone, subcutaneous injection once daily). Among the above-mentioned therapies, more similarities than differences exist; they are safe and usually well tolerated; they are equally expensive and effective in reducing the annual rate of relapses, but none of these agents can claim to prevent disability. High-dose IFN-β treatment showed superior relapse control and MRI stability compared to low-dose treatment in a systematic review of comparative studies.[68]. However, IFNs might cause side effects, including liver dysfunction, fatigue, thyroid disorders, inflammation at the injection site, headache, and flu-like symptoms [1,8,68].

Tailoring the treatment according to type of the disease (clinical course, relapsing or not), subgroup of MS (immunological), clinical activity, MRI activity, escalation of the intensity of treatment, the clinicians could escalate from first to second "line" treatment. Second-line DMT for MS is natalizumab (Tysabri; Elan/biogen Idec), a selective adhesion molecule inhibitor which reduces the migration of autoreactive TLs into the CNS by blocking the binding of very late antigen-4; it is generally recommended for patients who have had an insufficient response or intolerance to first-line treatment for MS. Switching to natalizumab or immunosuppressants in patients with breakthrough disease is effective in reducing clinical activity of relapsing MS [69]. However, the risk of developing progressive multifocal leukoencephalopathy (PML), an infection caused by the activation of the JC virus, with tropism for oligodendrocytes following natalizumab therapy, overshadows the benefits for some patients [7,70,71]. Until May 2010, more than 50 cases of PML have occurred in MS patients with natalizumab monotherapy. The risk of PML rises with duration of exposure to natalizumab [72].

Immunosuppressants (azathioprine, methotrexate), cytotoxic agents (mitoxantrone, cyclophosphamide) and chronic usage of corticosteroids continue to be a therapeutic option in patients with aggressive disease. The risk of secondary malignancies or severe adverse effects such as bone marrow toxicity-suppression, liver abnormalities (azathioprine, methotrexate) and renal toxicity and hypertension (cyclosporine) are well documented and place therapeutic laminations [73].

Combination therapies are based on additive immune effects of two distinct mechanisms of action eliciting a synergistic effect. Combination therapy of IFN-β with methyl-prednisolone IV or immunosupressants (methotrexate, cyclophosphamide, azathioprine, mitoxantrone) or glatiramer acetate with statins, mitoxantrone, minocycline have been tested in small clinical trials [1,7]. However, the usefulness of combination of IFNs and glatiramer acetate therapy in MS remains uncertain [74].

In PPMS there is no agent to alter the progression of the disease. A placebo-controlled study of methylprednisolone daily for five days followed by oral prednisone for a further four days reported beneficial effects for overall EDSS scores [75]. Emerging agents for RRMS that have shown some promise in MS include alemtuzumab, cladribine, daclizumab, dimethyl fumarate, laquinimod, minocycline, rituximab, statins, temsirolimus and teriflunomide [7,76]. More recently, six agents (alemtuzumab, BG00012, cladribine, fingolimod, laquinimod, teriflunomide) have completed phase 3 trials in RRMS. FDA committee in USA recommended fingolimod (trade name Gilenia), a synthetic analogue of the fungal sphingosine 1-phosphate (S1P) receptor agonist myriocin for the treatment of MS; it is the first oral drug to reduce relapses and delay disability progression in patients with relapsing forms of MS inhibiting lymphocytes to exit from lymphoid tissue, therefore it blocks the lymphocyte migration. Clinical trials of fingolimod have demonstrated side effects in treated patients including bradycardia, macular edema and visual blurring, CNS severe infections, liver toxicity and malignancies [77].

Epidemiological and experimental data suggest that vitamin D is involved in the pathogenesis of MS and may confer prevention and treatment of CIS and MS. Among other immunological properties, vitamin D increases Th2 cytokine production. Furthermore 1,25 dihydroxyvitamin D3 prevents the induction of EAE. Recommended daily dose of 400 IU of vitamin D reduces the risk of developing MS [7, 78].

Conventional drugs, including DMTs, various cytostatic regimens and steroids are unable to control the disease activity in a small group of patients with "malignant" MS. This group of patients could be offered aggressive therapies, such as high-dose immunosuppression followed by hematopoietic stem cell transplantation (HSCT). Bone marrow or peripheral blood HSCT has been proposed for the therapy of autoimmune diseases because of its immunosuppressive and immunomodulatory effects, and recapitulation of lymphocyte ontogeny may stabilize or improve the course of MS in some patients. A limited number of small studies conducted by using high-dose immuneablation and HSCT. A recent clinical trial of 85 patients treated by HSCT revealed that more than 60% of patients may benefit from this approach. Due to the perceived risks associated with HSCT, only patients with malignant MS who no longer benefit from more conventional therapies were enrolled; it is not a treatment for the general population of MS patients but only for selected cases that do not respond to standard therapies and worsen rapidly, i.e. in situations where benefits are expected to counterbalance morbidity and mortality risks [79,80]. Additional studies on the safety and efficacy of ongoing therapies such as antigen-specific therapies, neuroprotective therapy (e.g., glutamate receptor modulation), neural stem-cell transplantation and HSCT are needed [7].

Symptomatic Medications

Symptomatic treatment of MS is focused on the symptoms that arise by the disease and have a serious impact on the quality of life MS patients. Spasticity appears as stiffness, cramps, spasms or/and clonus. Mild spasticity at the beginning should be relieved by stretching exercises and physical therapy. Individual approach is required and includes muscle relaxants (such as tizanidine, baclofen, benzodiazepines (Valium) and anticonvulsants (gabapentin). In severe spasticity, intrathecal baclofen pump could be considered.

Fatigue occurs in 75 to 80% of MS patients. It appears to be multifactorial, with "primary" or disease-related factors involved, as well as "secondary" factors including comorbidities [81]. Physical and cooling therapy have been used. Additional pharmacological agents such as amantadine hydrochloride, modafinil and armodafinil have some efficacy.

Bladder dysfunction is a common problem for over 50% of MS patients. Bladder hypertonia is treated with anticholinergic drugs such as oxybutynin (Ditropan). Bladder-emptying regimen and intermittent catheterization may also be helpful for refractory incontinence.

Treatment for constipation includes high-fiber diet, increased fluid intake, daily exercise, and stool softeners. Rectal suppositories or enemas may be required occasionally. Managing bowel function was rated as having an impact equal to mobility difficulties on the quality of life of MS patients.

Sexual dysfunction may occur in men and women with MS and is caused by medications used for other symptoms such as antidepressants. Treatment is available for erectile dysfunction and female sexual dysfunction. Psychotherapy combined with antidepressants is an effective treatment for depression and anxiety [82].

Rehabilitation Programs

Patients with MS commonly experience poor postural control affecting mobility and/or cognitive impairment even in the early stages of the disease [83]; neurological abnormalities due to MS manifest themselves with a wide range of symptoms like the mentioned fatigue, numbness, paresthesiae, muscular weakness and spasticity, double vision, optic neuritis, ataxia, bladder control problems, dysphagia, dysarthria and cognitive dysfunction. These impairments can lead to relevant problems in carrying out activities of daily living. A range of therapies may be advised depending on what individual problems or disabilities the patients develop. Multidisciplinary rehabilitation approach improving the quality of life of MS patients is needed and includes [84]:

- Physiotherapy
- Supportive therapy
- Occupational therapy
- Speech therapy
- Cognitive therapy
- Psychotherapy
- Specialist nurse advice and support

References

[1] Compston A, Confavreux C, Lassman H, et al. *McAlpine's multiple sclerosis*. 4th ed. Edinburgh, Scotland: Churchill Livingstone, 2006.

[2] Kasper LH, Shoemaker J. Multiple sclerosis immunology: The healthy immune system vs the MS immune system. *Neurology* 2010;74 (Suppl 1):S2-8.

[3] McFarland HF, Martin R. Multiple sclerosis: a complicated picture of autoimmunity. *Nat Immunol* 2007;8:913-9.

[4] Sadovnick AD. European Charcot Foundation Lecture: the natural history of multiple sclerosis and gender. *J Neurol Sci* 2009;286:1-5.

[5] Vukusic S, Hutchinson M, Hours M, et al. Pregnancy and multiple sclerosis (the PRIMS study): clinical predictors of post-partum relapse. *Brain* 2004;127:1353-60.

[6] Lassmann H. Axonal and neuronal pathology in multiple sclerosis: what have we learnt from animal models. *Exp Neurol* 2010;225:2-8.

[7] Weiner HL. The challenge of multiple sclerosis: how do we cure a chronic heterogeneous disease? *Ann Neurol* 2009;65:239-48.

[8] Deretzi G, Kountouras J, Koutlas E, et al. Familial prevalence of autoimmune disorders in multiple sclerosis in Northern Greece. *Mult Scler* 2010;16:1091-101.

[9] International Multiple Sclerosis Genetics Consortium (IMSGC). IL12A, MPHOSPH9/CDK2AP1 and RGS1 are novel multiple sclerosis susceptibility loci. *Genes Immun* 2010;11:397-405.

[10] Beyeen AD, Adzemovic MZ, Ockinger J, et al. IL-22RA2 associates with multiple sclerosis and macrophage effector mechanisms in experimental neuroinflammation. *J Immunol* 2010;185:6883-90.

[11] McDowell TY, Amr S, Culpepper WJ, et al. Sun exposure, vitamin d and age at disease onset in relapsing multiple sclerosis. *Neuroepidemiology* 2011;36:39-45.

[12] Giovannoni G, Cutter GR, Lunemann J, et al. Infectious causes of multiple sclerosis. *Lancet Neurol* 2006;5:887-94.

[13] Serres S, Anthony DC, Jiang Y, et al. Systemic inflammatory response reactivates immune-mediated lesions in rat brain. *J Neurosci* 2009;29:4820-8.

[14] Ascherio A, Munger KL. 99th Dahlem conference on infection, inflammation and chronic inflammatory disorders: Epstein-Barr virus and multiple sclerosis: epidemiological evidence. *Clin Exp Immunol* 2010;160:120-4.

[15] Gavalas E, Kountouras J, Deretzi G, et al. *Helicobacter pylori* and multiple sclerosis. *J Neuroimmunol* 2007;188:187-9.

[16] Kountouras J, Gavalas E, Deretzi G, et al. *Helicobacter pylori* with or without its neutrophil-activating protein may be the common denominator associated with multiple sclerosis and neuromyelitis optica. *Mult Scler* 2010;16:376-7.

[17] Olson JK, Ercolini AM, Miller SD. A virus-induced molecular mimicry model ofmultiple sclerosis. *Curr Top Microbiol Immunol* 2005;296:39-53.

[18] Kurtzke JF, Heltberg A. Multiple sclerosis in the Faroe Islands: an epitome. *J Clin Epidemiol* 2001;54:1-22.

[19] Casiraghi C, Dorovini-Zis K, Horwitz MS. Epstein-Barr virus infection of human brain microvessel endothelial cells: a novel role in multiple sclerosis. *J Neuroimmunol* 2011;230:173-7.

[20] Li W, Minohara M, Piao H, et al. Association of anti-*Helicobacter pylori* neutrophil-activating protein antibody response with anti-aquaporin-4 autoimmunity in Japanese patients with multiple sclerosis and neuromyelitis optica. *Mult Scler* 2009;15:1411-21.

[21] Kountouras J, Tsolaki M, Gavalas E, et al. Relationship between *Helicobacter pylori* infection and Alzheimer disease. *Neurology* 2006;66:938-40.

[22] Deretzi G, Kountouras J, Grigoriadis N et al. From the "little brain" gastrointestinal infection to the "big brain" neuroinflammation: a proposed fast axonal transport pathway involved in multiple sclerosis. *Med Hypotheses* 2009;73:781-7.

[23] Kountouras J. *Helicobacter pylori*: an intruder involved in conspiring glaucomatous neuropathy. *Br J Ophthalmol* 2009;93:1413-5.

[24] Candelario-Jalil E, Taheri S, Yang Y, et al. Cyclooxygenase inhibition limitsblood–brain barrier disruption following intracerebral injection of tumor necrosis factor-alpha in the rat. *J Pharmacol Exp Ther* 2007;323:488-98.

[25] Supajatura V, Ushio H, Wada A, et al. Cutting edge: VacA, a vacuolatingcytotoxin of *Helicobacter pylori*, directly activates mast cells for migration and production of proinflammatory cytokines. *J Immunol* 2002;168:2603-7.

[26] Kountouras J, Zavos C, Diamantidis MD, et al. A concept of *Helicobacter pylori* and stress-secreted mast cells' potential involvement in brain metastases. *J Neuroimmunol* 2009;209:121-2.

[27] Theoharides TC, Rozniecki JJ, Sahagian G, et al. Impact of stress and mast cells on brain metastases. *J Neuroimmunol* 2008;205:1-7.

[28] Wang YH, Wu JJ, Lei HY. When *Helicobacter pylori* invades and replicates in the cells. *Autophagy* 2009;5:540-2.

[29] Lassmann H, Brück W, Lucchinetti CF. The immunopathology of multiple sclerosis: an overview. *Brain Pathol* 2007;17:210-8.

[30] Lucchinetti, C, Brück W, Parisi J, et al. Heterogeneity of multiple sclerosis lesions: implications for the pathogenesis of demyelination. *Ann Neurol* 2000;47:707-17.

[31] Glass CK, Saijo K, Winner B, et al. Mechanisms underlying inflammation in neurodegeneration. *Cell* 2010;140:918-34.

[32] Costantino CM, Baecher-Allan C, Hafler DA. Multiple sclerosis and regulatory T cells. *J Clin Immunol* 2008;28:697-706.

[33] Schneider-Hohendorf T, Stenner MP, Weidenfeller C, et al. Regulatory T cells exhibit enhanced migratory characteristics, a feature impaired in patients with multiple sclerosis. *Eur J Immunol* 2010;40:3581-90.

[34] Town T, Nikolic V, Tan J. The microglial ''activation'' continuum: from innate to adaptive responses. *J Neuroinflammation* 2005;2:24.

[35] Buntinx M, Moreels M, Vandenabeele F, et al. Cytokine-induced cell death in human oligodendroglial cell lines: I. Synergistic effects of IFN-gamma and TNF-alpha on apoptosis. *J Neurosci Res* 2004;76:834-45.

[36] Kountouras J, Zavos C, Chatzopoulos D. Induction of apoptosis as a proposed pathophysiological link between glaucoma and *Helicobacter pylori* infection. *Med Hypotheses* 2004;62:378-81.

[37] Van Horssen J, Witte ME, Schreibelt G, et al. Radical changes in multiple sclerosis pathogenesis. *Biochim Biophys Acta* 2011;1812:141-50.

[38] Ray A, Mann MK, Basu S, et al. A case for regulatory B cells in controlling the severity of autoimmune-mediated inflammation in experimental autoimmune encephalomyelitis and multiple sclerosis. *J Neuroimmunol* 2011;230:1-9.

[39] Magliozzi R, Howell OW, Reeves C, et al. A gradient of neuronal loss and meningeal inflammation in multiple sclerosis. *Ann Neurol* 2010;68:477-93.

[40] Barnett MH, Prineas JW. Relapsing and remitting multiple sclerosis: pathology of the newly forming lesion. *Ann Neurol* 2004;55:458-68.

[41] Trapp BD, Peterson J, Ransohoff RM, et al. Axonal transection in the lesions of multiple sclerosis. *N Engl J Med* 1998;338:278-285.

[42] Schirmer L, Antel JP, Brück W, et al. Axonal loss and neurofilament phosphorylation changes accompany lesion development and clinical progression in multiple sclerosis. *Brain Pathol* 2011;21:428-40.

[43] Kirov I, Patil V, Babb J, et al. MR spectroscopy indicates diffuse multiple sclerosis activity during remission. *J Neurol Neurosurg Psychiatry* 2009;80:1330-6.

[44] Calabrese M, Rinaldi F, Grossi P, et al. Basal ganglia and frontal/parietal cortical atrophy is associated with fatigue in relapsing-remitting multiple sclerosis. *Mult Scler* 2010;16:1220-8.
[45] Compston A, Coles A. "Multiple sclerosis". *Lancet* 2008;372:1502-17.
[46] Tremlett H, Zhao Y, Rieckmann P, et al. New perspectives in the natural history of multiple sclerosis. *Neurology* 2010;74:2004-15.
[47] Montalban X, Tintoré M, Swanton J, et al. MRI criteria for MS in patients with clinically isolated syndromes. *Neurology* 2010;74:427-34.
[48] Koch M, Kingwell E, Rieckmann P, et al. The natural history of secondary progressive multiple sclerosis. UBC MS Clinic Neurologists. *J Neurol Neurosurg Psychiatry* 2010;81:1039-44.
[49] Glad SB, Nyland H, Aarseth JH, et al. How long can you keep working with benign multiple sclerosis? *J Neurol Neurosurg Psychiatry* 2011;82:78-82.
[50] Venkateswaran S, Banwell B. Pediatric multiple sclerosis. *Neurologist* 2010;16:92-105.
[51] Awad A, Stüve O. Multiple sclerosis in the elderly patient. *Drugs Aging* 2010;27:283-94.
[52] Stadelmann C, Brück W. Lessons from the neuropathology of atypical forms of multiple sclerosis. *Neurol Sci* 2004;25(Suppl 4):S319-22.
[53] McDonald WI, Compston A, Edan G, et al. Recommended diagnostic criteria for multiple sclerosis: guidelines from the International Panel on the diagnosis of multiple sclerosis. *Ann Neurol* 2001;50:121-7.
[54] Polman CH, Reingold SC, Banwell B, et al. Diagnostic criteria for multiple sclerosis: 2010 revisions to the McDonald criteria. *Ann Neurol 2011*;69:292-302.
[55] Kurtzke JF. Rating neurologic impairment in multiple sclerosis: an expanded disability status scale (EDSS). *Neurology* 1983;33:1444-52.
[56] Sormani MP, Stubinski B, Cornelisse P, et al. Magnetic resonance active lesions as individual-level surrogate for relapses in multiple sclerosis. *Mult Scler* 2011;17:541-9.
[57] Rovira A, Swanton J, Tintoré M, et al. A single, early magnetic resonance imaging study in the diagnosis of multiple sclerosis. *Arch Neurol* 2009;66:587-9.
[58] Link H, Huang YM. Oligoclonal bands in multiple sclerosis cerebrospinal fluid: an update on methodology and clinical usefulness. *J Neuroimmunol* 2006;180:17-28.
[59] Schäffler N, Köpke S, Winkler L, et al. Accuracy of diagnostic tests in multiple sclerosis - a systematic review. *Acta Neurol Scand* 2011;124:151-64.
[60] Whiting P, Harbord R, Main C, et al. Accuracy of magnetic resonance imaging for the diagnosis of multiple sclerosis: systematic review. *BMJ* 2006;332:875-4.
[61] Miller DH, Weinshenker BG, Filippi M, et al. Differential diagnosis of suspected multiple sclerosis: a consensus approach. *Mult Scler* 2008;14:1157-74.
[62] Arnson Y, Shoenfeld Y, Alon E, et al. The antiphospholipid syndrome as a neurological disease. *Semin Arthritis Rheum* 2010;40:97-108.
[63] Brinar VV, Poser CM. The spectrum of disseminated encephalomyelitis. *Clin Neurol Neurosurg* 2006;108:2295-310.
[64] Weinshenker BG, Wingerchuk DM, Vukusic S, et al. Neuromyelitis optica IgG predicts relapse after longitudinal extensive transverse myelitis. *Ann Neurol* 2006;59:566-9.

[65] Miller DM, Weinstock GB, Bethoux F et al. A meta-analysis of methylprednisolone in recovery from multiple sclerosis exacerbations. *Mult Scler* 2000;6:267-73.
[66] Thrower B. Relapse Management in Multiple Sclerosis. *Neurologist* 2009;15:1-5.
[67] Freedman MS. Improving long-term follow-up studies of immunomodulatory therapies. *Neurology* 2011;76(1 Suppl 1):S35-8.
[68] Oliver BJ, Kohli E, Kasper LH. Interferon therapy in relapsing-remitting multiple sclerosis: A systematic review and meta-analysis of the comparative trials. J *Neurol Sci* 2011;302:96-105.
[69] Castillo-Trivino T, Mowry EM, Gajofatto A, et al. Switching multiple sclerosis patients with breakthrough disease to second-line therapy. *PLoS One* 2011;6:e16664.
[70] Marriott JJ, O'Connor PW. Lessons learned from long-term multiple sclerosis treatment trials. *Mult Scler* 2010;16:1028-30.
[71] Gajofatto A, Bacchetti P, Grimes B, et al. Switching first-line disease-modifying therapy after failure: impact on the course of relapsing-remitting multiple sclerosis. *Mult Scler* 2008;15:50-8.
[72] Warnke C, Menge T, Hartung HP, et al. Natalizumab and progressive multifocal leukoencephalopathy: what are the causal factors and can it be avoided? *Arch Neurol* 2010;67:923-30.
[73] Kieseier BC, Jeffery DR. Chemotherapeutics in the treatment of multiple sclerosis. *Ther Adv Neurol Disord* 2010;3:277-91.
[74] Conway D, Cohen JA. Combination therapy in multiple sclerosis. *Lancet Neurol* 2010;9:299-308.
[75] Bates D. Treatment effects of immunomodulatory therapies at different stages of multiple sclerosis in short-term trials. *Neurology* 2011;76(1 Suppl 1):S14-25.
[76] Cohen JA. Emerging therapies for relapsing multiple sclerosis. *Arch Neurol* 2009;66:821-8.
[77] Cohen JA, Barkhof F, Comi G, et al. Oral fingolimod or intramuscular interferon for relapsing multiple sclerosis. *N Eng J Med* 2010;362:402-15.
[78] Smolders J. Vitamin d and multiple sclerosis: correlation, causality, and controversy. *Autoimmune Dis* 2010;2011:629538.
[79] Havrdova E. Aggressive multiple sclerosis-is there a role for stem cell transplantation? *J Neurol* 2005;252:Suppl 3:iii34-7.
[80] Fassas A, Mancardi GL. Autologous hemopoietic stem cell transplantation for multiple sclerosis: is it worthwhile? *Autoimmunity* 2008;41:601-10.
[81] Kaminska M, Kimoff RJ, Schwartzman K, et al. Sleep disorders and fatigue in multiple sclerosis: Evidence for association and interaction. *J Neurol Sci* 2011;302:7-13.
[82] Thompson AJ, Toosy AT, Ciccarelli O. Pharmacological management of symptoms in multiple sclerosis: current approaches and future directions. *Lancet Neurol* 2010;9:1182-99.
[83] Kalron A, Dvir Z, Achiron A. Effect of a cognitive task on postural control in patients with a clinically isolated syndrome suggestive of multiple sclerosis. *Eur J Phys Rehabil Med* 2011 Feb 9. [Epub ahead of print].
[84] Simmons RD. Life issues in multiple sclerosis. *Nat Rev Neurol* 2010;6:603-10.

In: Multiple Sclerosis
Editor: E. Scholz and C. Müller, pp. 81-96

ISBN 978-1-61324-848-5

Chapter IV

Epstein-Barr Virus and Multiple Sclerosis

Costanza Casiraghi and Marc S. Horwitz*
Department of Microbiology and Immunology, The University British Columbia, Vancouver, British Columbia, Canada

Abstract

Multiple sclerosis (MS) is an immune-mediated disease of the central nervous system that leads to myelin loss and progressive disability. The causes of MS are still unknown but the disease process is likely triggered by an environmental factor(s) in genetically susceptible individuals. Several different viruses have been identified as possible MS triggers but increasing evidence strongly associates Epstein-Barr virus (EBV) to MS. Epidemiological findings show that EBV infection, especially if accompanied by mononucleosis, greatly increases MS risk. Other relevant findings include the correlation between disease onset and the titer of anti-EBV antibodies in the serum. Dysregulated EBV specific T cells responses have been detected in MS, suggesting that MS patients might have a decreased ability to control EBV replication and there is also evidence of cross-reactivity between EBV antigens and myelin. The main site of EBV latency is the B cell compartment and B cell depletion therapies have been recently shown to strongly reduce disease activity in relapsing-remitting MS. Intriguingly EBV positive B cell follicles have been found in the brain of MS patients. Further, EBV has been shown to infect cell types other than B cells and these could play a role in MS pathogenesis. Despite all these findings, it is still unclear how EBV triggers MS. In this review we will summarize past literature and discuss possible mechanisms that EBV is exploiting to trigger MS.

* Correspondence should be addressed to: Marc S. Horwitz. Department of Microbiology and Immunology, 2350 Health Sciences Mall, Vancouver, BC, Canada, V6T1Z3, email: mhorwitz@interchange.ubc.ca.

Introduction

Multiple Sclerosis (MS) is a chronic inflammatory disease of the central nervous system (CNS) that leads to myelin disruption and progressive disability. MS is believed to be triggered by environmental factors in genetically susceptible individuals but the etiology is still unknown. Myelin damage is thought to be mediated by autoreactive T cells. These T cells are able to cross the blood-brain barrier (BBB), recognize myelin epitopes and produce pro-inflammatory mediators that recruit a second wave of immune cells into the CNS. It is still not clear what is the first event that triggers myelin recognition, BBB breach and T cell entry into the CNS [Sospedra and Martin 2005].

A number of different viruses have been implicated as etiologic agents of MS since its first description. Jean-Martin Charcot, a French neurologist that first described and named the disease in 1868, related infections with disease onset in some patients [Clanet 2008]. Pierre Marie, a former student of Charcot, postulated that the disease was caused by an infection [Burks et al. 2000]. In the past 20 years, increasing evidence has indicated Epstein-Barr virus (EBV) as a potential trigger of MS. EBV is a herpesvirus that infects 90% of the population and it is usually acquired during childhood. If infection occurs during adolescence or adulthood, EBV causes mononucleosis. The virus establishes life-long latency in B cells and epithelial cells [Kieff and Rickinson 2007]. In this review we will summarize the findings that implicate EBV infection in MS pathogenesis and discuss possible new mechanism exploited by EBV to trigger MS.

The Development of a Hypothesis from 1970 to 2000

The first observations of a link between EBV and MS date back in the '70 and '80. In 1979, Fraser and colleagues noticed that lymphoid-cell lines (i.e. B cells transformed by EBV) are established more easily with lymphocytes isolated from patients with clinically active MS than with those from healthy donors. The authors recognized that: "even if there is no primary role for EBV in the immunology of MS, a secondary role of reactivated EBV in its pathogenesis should be considered" [Fraser 1979]. Later, Craig and colleagues published a series of articles in which they demonstrated that T cells from MS patients fail to suppress EBV transformed cells whereas all lymphocytes cultures from control (except those from seronegative and cord blood donors) are able to suppress EBV immortalized cells. They also found that MS patients have reduced numbers of CD8+ T cells and higher ratio of CD4+/CD8+ T cells [Craig et al. 1983,1985 and 1988].

During the same years, other papers were published showing increased EBV seropositivity and increased anti-EBV antibody titers among MS cohorts [Sumaya et al. 1980; Bray et al. 1983; Myhr et al. 1998]. Interestingly, the prevalence of herpes simplex virus (HSV), cytomegalovirus (CMV), varicella zoster virus (VZV), rubella and mumps infections in these cohorts did not differ between MS patients and controls. Moreover, according to a case-control study, MS patients reporting of having had infectious mononucleosis before the age of 18 years, have an increased relative risk of multiple sclerosis [Martin et al. 1993]. The authors of this article pointed out that: "the pathogenesis of multiple sclerosis may involve an age-dependent host response to Epstein-Barr virus infection". To further corroborate this theory, immigrant studies suggested that the risk of acquiring MS is determined by the area of residence during the first 15-18 years of life: people moving from a high risk to a low risk area after childhood retain the MS risk of their former area of residence. So, people living in an area where EBV is acquired during childhood and then moving to an area where EBV is more often acquired during/after adolescence would have a reduced risk of developing MS if compared to people that spent the first 15-18 years of their lives in areas in which EBV infection occurs later in life. [Warner and Carp 1981; 1988]. There are also striking similarities between MS and mononucleosis prevalence: they both follow the same latitude gradient and affect people with high socio-economic status [Warner and Carp 1981].

Finally, evidence of molecular mimicry between EBV and myelin antigen was demonstrated through a series of articles. Wucherpfennig and colleagues showed that three T cells clones isolated from MS patients and specific for myelin basic protein (MBP) can be also activated by both bacterial and viral peptides, including one EBV DNA polymerase peptide [Wucherpfennig et al. 1995]. Additionally, anti-EBV antibodies were found to be cross-reactive for neuroglial cells epitopes [Vaughan et al. 1996] and transaldolase, a protein expressed in olygodendrocytes [Esposito et al. 1999].

Association between EBV and MS in Epidemiological Studies

Early studies identified increased prevalence of EBV seropositivity among MS patients. Ascherio and colleagues reviewed eight studies [Ascherio and Munch 2000], including 1,005 cases and 1,060 controls, demonstrating that EBV seroprevalence among MS patients is virtually 100%, whereas it is 95-85% among the general population. More compelling results came subsequently from MS pediatric cohorts. In fact, EBV seropositivity is lower in children than in the adult population and differences in EBV seroprevalence in MS pediatric cases against controls are even more striking than in adults. The first study was conducted in 2004 [Alotaibi et al. 2004]: 30 pediatric MS patients were analyzed for the presence of antibodies against EBV and other herpesviruses (CMV, HSV and VZV) and they were compared with 90 age-matched emergency department controls and 53 healthy controls. EBV infection was detected in 83% of pediatric MS patients and in 42% of controls. Importantly seropositivity for other herpesviruses did not differ between the groups. Other studies followed with similar findings: 147 pediatric MS cases showed 98% EBV seropositivity, compared to 72% EBV seropositive age-matched controls [Pohl et al. 2006]; 86% of children with MS and 64% of healthy children were found seropositive for EBV in a large Canadian study enrolling 137 cases and 96 controls matched by age and geographical region. These two cohorts did not differ in seroprevalence of other viruses analyzed, thus confirming results from other studies [Banwell et al. 2007].

Additionally, EBV seropositivity and history of mononucleosis further increases the risk of developing MS [Nielsen et al. 2008; Ramagopalan et al. 2009; Handel et al. 2010; Levin et al. 2010]. A large Canadian study analyzed over 14,000 MS cases and 7,600 spouse controls asking about history of measles, mumps, rubella, varicella and infectious mononucleosis.

They found no differences between the groups except for mononucleosis: 699 cases and 165 controls indicated a history of infectious mononucleosis [Ramagopalan et al. 2009]. Another study showed that mononucleosis history and the human leukocyte antigen HLA-DRB1*15, both MS risk factors, increase MS risk in synergy. Individuals that never had mononucleosis but carry the allele DRB1*15 have a 2.4-fold increased MS risk. In contrast, in people with mononucleosis history, DRB1*15 is associated with a 7.0-fold increased MS risk. These data, combined with previous results, demonstrated that a person that carries DRB1*15 allele with a history of mononucleosis, has a 10-fold increased risk of MS compared with a person who is carrying DRB1*15 and never had mononucleosis [Nielsen et al. 2008]. Moreover, a review of previous published articles about the link between MS and mononucleosis, including over 19,000 cases and 16,000 controls, showed that MS risk is strongly associated with mononucleosis with a relative risk of 2.17 ($p=10^{-54}$) [Handel et al. 2010]. Another recent interesting study showed that MS risk increases if EBV seroconversion occurs. The authors studied 305 individuals who developed MS and 610 matched controls. To determine EBV infection, they measured anti-EBV antibody titers in serial blood samples collected before MS diagnosis among cases and, on matched dates, among controls. They found that all EBV negative cases converted into EBV positive before MS onset. On the other hand only 35.7% of controls seroconverted in the same period of time [Levin et al. 2010].

EBV Strains in MS Patients

The prevalence of EBV infection is very high in adults that never developed MS. So it is conceivable that MS patients are infected by a particular EBV strain that is able to cause MS. Only few article in the last years have addressed this question. In 2008, Lindsey and colleagues sequenced EBV using blood collected from MS patients and healthy controls. They sequenced EBV latent membrane protein-1 (LMP-1) because variations in this gene are associated with lymphoproliferative diseases. Different LMP-1 sequences were isolated from both cases and controls but there was no difference between the groups [Lindsey et al. 2008]. Similar results were obtained in a subsequent study that sequenced the N- and C-terminus regions of EBNA-1 and, again, LMP-1. EBNA-1 was chosen because anti-EBNA-1 antibody titer is associated with MS risk; LMP-1 because is able to activate B cells and immortalize them. Again, no differences were detected between cases and controls [Simon et al. 2010].

Another group sequenced EBNA-1 and BRRF-2 because of their ability to induce dysregulated immune responses in MS patients. Different polymorphisms were identified in both genes, in both cases and controls. A couple of SNPs were found to occur slightly more frequently in MS patients, but the study was not conclusive [Brennan et al. 2010]. More studies with larger numbers of cases and controls are likely needed to better address this type of question.

EBV Replication Control and Reactivation in MS Patients

Another mechanism that EBV could exploit to trigger MS is the ability to replicate better or reactivate more often in MS patients. This frequent reactivation could constantly stimulate the immune system leading to impairments in the maintenance of peripheral tolerance. Serological and genetic markers of EBV infection and reactivation were analyzed monthly for one year on 19 MS patients. Patients with clinical symptoms due to progression or relapses have frequent EBV reactivation and EBV genome is detected in 100% of these cases but in none of the MS patients with stable diseases. This was confirmed also through serological analysis. On the other hand, only 17% of controls showed EBV reactivation [Wandinger et al. 2000]. These data were partially confirmed by another study that measured EBV RNA and DNA levels in peripheral blood leukocytes (PBMCs) from cases and controls using quantitative PCR. There was no significant difference between the two groups, but paired samples showed EBV increase before and during relapses [Lindsey et al. 2009]. EBV plasma viral loads were also measured in a small group of MS patients and controls in another study. In this case, the authors did not find any difference between MS patients and control [Wagner et al. 2004]. Discrepancies in these studies maybe due to the small numbers of cases-controls analyzed, to the different type of starting material (plasma, blood or PBMCs) and different methodology (PCR or serology) employed to detect EBV reactivation.

EBV Humoral Responses in MS Patients

High antibody titers, called oligoclonal bands (OCB), are found in the cerebrospinal fluid (CSF) of MS patients. Their presence is used as diagnostic criteria for MS [Sospedra and Martin 2005]. The specificity of these antibodies is still largely unknown but some groups have investigated the possibility that they are specific for EBV proteins. In one of the early articles, OCB were found to be enriched in antibodies specific for EBV proteins, especially EBNA-1, in a subset of MS patients [Rand et al. 1998 & 2000]. Following investigations detected EBV reactivity along with reactivity against other herpesviruses; or did not find any reactivity; or found the same EBV reactivity in MS and other neurological inflammatory diseases [Pohl et al. 2009; Jafari et al. 2010; Franciotta et al. 2010]. This indicates that EBV humoral response in the CSF is maybe only part of the multispecific antibody production in MS that targets different neurotropic viruses.

On the other hand, studies on sera samples have produced more consistent results. In fact, patients affected by MS show a dysregulated humoral immune response against EBV in the serum both before the onset and during the course of the disease. This observation was first made in 2001, when Ascherio and colleagues analyzed blood samples collected before MS onset and they showed that MS patients have higher serum titers of anti-EBV antibodies but not anti-CMV antibodies. EBV antibodies were also found elevated in 126 MS cases after disease onset when compared to their matched controls [Ascherio et al. 2001]. Following studies confirmed and further strengthened these results. Prospectively collected serum samples were analyzed for EBV EBNA-1, CMV, HHV-6, HSV, VZV and measles reactivity.

Only high activity to EBNA-1 significantly increases the risk of MS and it is more pronounced five years before onset of clinical symptoms [Sundstrom et al. 2004]. Also Levin and colleagues found that the strongest predictor of MS is anti-EBNA-1 antibody titer. In their cohort of MS patients and controls, individuals that develop the disease have serum EBNA-1 antibody titers similar to those of controls before the age of 20 years, but the titer increases of 2-3 fold after the age of 25. Titers of antibodies against others EBV proteins (VCA and EBNA-2) or CMV did not differ between the groups [Levin et al. 2005]. Another study determined that EBNA-1 antibodies start to be elevated in comparison with matched controls even up to fifteen to twenty years before development of clinical symptoms. The antibody titer remains then elevated until clinical manifestations occur [DeLorenze et al. 2006]. Increased EBNA-1 antibodies titers are also found in pediatric MS cohorts [Lunemann et al. 2008a] and in MS patients when compared to healthy siblings raised in the same family household [Comabella et al. 2010]. Interestingly, these findings have been shown to be specific for MS. EBNA-1 antibodies levels are not increased in the CSF or in the serum of patients suffering from other inflammatory and non-inflammatory neurological diseases [Nociti et al. 2010]. Overall, these results indicate that elevated IgG responses against EBNA-1 are strongly linked to MS onset and they can predict conversion to MS. This has been observed in a study that analyzed humoral immune responses against EBV and other viruses (HHV-6, CMV and measles) in patients with clinically isolated syndrome (CIS) to assess if viral antibody titers can predict conversion to MS. EBNA-1 IgG titers were the only that correlate with number of brain lesions, disability severity and predict conversion to MS according to McDonald criteria [Lunemann et al. 2010].

Furthermore higher anti EBNA-1 antibody titers are associated with increased presence of new MS lesions in the brain as detected with magnetic resonance (MRI) [Farrell et al. 2009], with increased disability and increased loss of brain volume and grey matter atrophy [Zivadinov et al. 2009].

Finally, other groups tried to assess if antibodies against other EBV protein were elevated before MS onset. For example, Massa and colleagues chose to measure anti-BZLF-1 antibody titers because they predict another EBV-induced disease, nasopharyngeal carcinoma. They again found increased EBNA-1 antibodies titers but no differences on BZLF-1 titers between cases and controls [Massa et al. 2007]. Increased immune responses against EBV EBNA-1 in MS (a marker of EBV latency) and lack of association with lytic-late EBV proteins responses (like BZLF-1 or VCA) suggest a limited role of viral reactivation in MS pathogenesis.

EBV T Cell Responses in MS Patients

Molecular mimicry between EBV and myelin antigens has been demonstrated for the first time in the 1995 with the isolation of a cross-reactive T cell clone from a MS patient [Wucherpfenning et al. 1995]. The structure of this cross-reactive T cell-receptor (TCR), bound to two different MHC allele/peptide complexes, was later solved, with X-ray crystallography. The authors showed that this TCR can bind and recognize with high degree of structural equivalence two different MHC alleles/peptide complexes: DRB1*1501 presenting a myelin antigen and DRB5*0101 presenting an EBV antigen. Intriguingly both MHC alleles are associated with MS risk [Lang et al. 2002].

Cross-reactive T cells can be also detected in the CSF fluid of MS patients, indicating that lymphocytes can gain access to the CNS: CD4+ T cells specific for both an EBV polymerase peptide and a myelin basic protein peptide were in fact isolated from two MS patients [Holmoy et al. 2004].

Another mechanism that EBV could exploit to trigger MS is through an increased or decreased EBV specific CD8 or CD4 response. An increased EBV specific immunity with more cytotoxic activity or more IFN-γ production can lead to a bystander activation of auto-reactive T cells. On the other hand, a decreased T cell immunity against EBV could lead to frequent viral reactivation and chronic stimulation of the immune system with loss of peripheral tolerance. Different studies have shown that both scenarios could be possible.

CD8 T cells responses against two EBV antigens HLA-B7 restricted (EBNA-3 and LMP-2) have been found increased in MS patients if compared to healthy controls. CD8 responses to these epitopes were measured by an ELISPOT assay detecting IFN-γ production. Responses to a CMV immunodominant peptide did not differ between cases and controls [Hollsberg et al. 2003]. Different results were obtained in another article in which the authors tested the frequency of CD8 T cells specific for other HLA-B7 restricted EBV peptides (EBNA-1, BZLF-1 and BBLF-2/3), using again an ELISPOT assay. The authors did not find any significant difference between MS patients and healthy controls [Gronen et al. 2006]. This might be due to the fact that different peptides were tested. On the other hand, increased frequency of EBV specific CD8 T cells in MS patients was again confirmed by another group with a different experimental approach: T cells from cases and controls were incubated with autologous EBV-transformed B cells and then stained for IFN-γ production [Cepok et al. 2005]. Additionally it has been demonstrated that EBV specific CD8 responses are more elevated at MS onset and then tend to decrease over time. Jilek and colleagues analyzed EBV specific CD8 T cells IFN-γ production in patients with CIS, relapsing-remitting MS (RR-MS), secondary progressive MS (SP-MS) and patients with other neurological disease. CIS patients have the highest frequency of EBV specific CD8 and this frequency decreases after one year [Jilek at al. 2008]. Another group confirmed these results detecting higher numbers of EBV specific CD8 T cell in the CSF of MS patients at early disease stage using a CFSE-based cytotoxic assay [Jaquiery et al. 2010a]. Moreover EBV specific CD8 T cells isolated from MS patients express higher levels of both IFN-γ and IL-4 [Jaquiery et al. 2010b]. This might indicate that EBV has an important role as initial disease trigger. The results of these studies are specific for MS and EBV infection only, since dysregulation of EBV immunity is not detected in both inflammatory and non-inflammatory neurological diseases. Additionally CMV specific responses are equivalent between MS patients and controls.

All these studies point in favor of the hypothesis that MS patients have an increased and dysregulated immune response against EBV that could lead to bystander activation of an autoimmune response. On the other hand, as mentioned above, there is also evidence that MS patients may have a decreased EBV specific T cells response, leading to impairment in EBV infection control. Pender and colleagues analyzed the frequency of PBMCs that produce IFN-γ when exposed to autologous EBV infected B cells isolated from 34 MS patients and 34 EBV positive controls. They found decreased CD8 T cell responses against transformed B cells in MS patients. They also showed that this impairment was not due to decreased HLA expression on B cells or a primary defect in the function of the CD8 compartment [Pender at al. 2009]. A similar result was found by another group that detected decreased EBV specific

CD8 responses in MS patients using the same experimental approach of Pender and colleagues [Lindsey and Hatfield, 2010].

Finally other published work analyzed EBV specific CD4 T cells responses, especially EBNA-1 specific response, since MS patients have dysregulated antibody response against EBNA-1 and EBNA-1 specific CD4 T cells have been shown to be important for EBV control in healthy subjects. A first study, using over fifty overlapping peptides covering the C-terminal domain of EBNA-1, showed increased frequency of EBNA-1 specific CD4+ memory T cells in MS patients. These cells are also able to proliferate more and produce more IFN-γ. T cell responses against other EBV latent and lytic immunodominant peptides and CMV epitopes did not differ between cases and controls. While CD4 T cells from controls are able to recognize a restricted central part of the EBNA-1

C-terminal domain, T cells from MS patients recognized epitopes present in the whole domain. [Lunemann et al. 2006]. A second article further characterized EBNA-1 specific CD4 T cells as central memory Th1 helper precursors and Th1 polarized effector memory T cells. Intriguingly these T cells are able to cross-recognize myelin epitopes more frequently. Additionally myelin cross-reactive CD4 cells are able to produce both IFN-γ and IL-2; whereas EBNA-1 specific, non cross-reactive CD4 cells are producing IFN-γ only [Lunemann et al. 2008b]. This IL-2 and IFN-γ polyfunctional phenotype is typical of persistent infections and gives credit to the theory that both molecular mimicry and bystander activation, through dysregulated cytokine production, can have a role in MS onset.

EBV Infection in the MS Brain

Since MS was first described in 1868, different investigators postulated that myelin damage was caused by a virus infecting the CNS. As soon as EBV was implicated in MS pathogenesis, the quest to find EBV in MS plaques started. Few negative articles were initially published [Hilton et al. 1994; Opsahal and Kennedy 2007]. The main technique used to detect EBV infection in these articles was in situ-hybridization using probes against EBER, an EBV RNA transcript expressed during latency. RNA preservation was tested using control probes specific for housekeeping genes and EBV positive lymphoma tissue was used as positive control. The authors recognized some caveats of this approach: RNA degradation was present in some of the samples analyzed due to long formalin fixation and the majority of lesion analyzed were chronic lesions, not representative of the initial stages of the disease [Opsahal and Kennedy 2007]. Another group employed a highly sensitive PCR approach, able to detect one EBV positive cell, to detect EBV infection in paraffin embedded active demyelinating MS lesion collected at autopsy. All the lesions analyzed with this approach tested negative for EBV infection [Morrè at al. 2001].

In 2007, Aloisi's group published for the first time evidence that EBV is able indeed to infect the MS brain [Serafini et al. 2007]. Eight cases of SP-MS with ectopic follicles in the meninges and B cells/plasmacells infiltration in the white matter were analyzed. Additionally brain specimens from 12 cases of RR-MS and 2 cases of acute MS were stained. Ectopic follicles are lymphoid structures in the meninges and have germinal centre features: they are composed of CD20+ cells surrounded by stromal/dendritic cells. Moreover CXCL13 expression, proliferation and differentiation of B cells into plasmacells are detected in the follicles. Both intrameningeal ectopic follicles and perivascular cuffs of acute and chronic active white matter lesions stain positive for EBER through in situ-hybridization. The author termed the brain specimen from these MS patients as "EBV high". Lower levels of EBV infection are also detected in all the other brain samples analyzed (termed as "EBV low") except one. The negative brain sample was also negative for B cells infiltrations, while in the EBV low cases, EBV infection was present in B cells and plasmacells scattered in the parenchyma or close to the perivascular area. Brain section of other inflammatory and non-inflammatory CNS diseases tested negative for EBV infection. Immunofluorescence and immunohistochemistry for different EBV proteins showed that only latency proteins are generally expressed. But, in some EBV high cases and in acute MS cases also lytic EBV protein are detected, mainly in plasmacells, indicating EBV reactivation. EBV replication is likely abortive since viral glycoprotein expression is not detected. EBV high cases present with CD8+ T cells that are producing perforin and IFN-γ and they are concomitant with infected B cells. This indicates that the presence of a lytic EBV infection in the CNS is recruiting pro-inflammatory immune cells, both T cells and APCs to counteract the infection. This response could start a pro-inflammatory loop with initial myelin damage, recruitment and bystander activation of myelin autoreactive T cells. A second article by Aloisi's group, that further confirms EBV infection, employed laser–capture microdissection to isolate and analyze a fraction of the tissue of interest [Serafini et al. 2010]. Intrameningeal B cells follicles areas and surrounding normal appearing brain areas are harvested, RNA is extracted and EBV cDNA is enriched with a pre-amplification reverse transcription: expression of LMP-1 and LMP-2A, two EBV proteins involved in survival and maturation of B cells, are expressed in B cells and they are not detected in any other normal areas of the brain analyzed. High levels of BAFF expression are also detected in EBV infected B cells in acute lesions and ectopic B cells follicles. BAFF is a B cell activator involved in B cell responses independent of T cells; intriguingly overexpression of BAFF leads to autoimmunity in mice and loss of B cell tolerance. The expression of this factor in EBV infected B cells could contribute to the persistence of infected cells in the CNS.

Other groups were not able to reproduce these findings and they did not find evidence of EBV infection in the MS brain [Sargsyan et al. 2010; Willis et al. 2009; Peferoen et al. 2010]. Willis and colleagues analyzed 24 MS brains and did not find EBV infection in a first set of 12 cases. They employed in situ hybridization, immunohistochemistry and real-time PCR for genomic EBV or EBER. In a second set of 12 cases, they detect low levels of EBV through PCR only in a couple of meningeal samples. Peferoen and colleagues analyzed specimens from 94 patients with MS, including 12 patients screened in the Serafini et al. article. They used in situ hybridization for EBER and immunohistochemistry for latent and lytic EBV proteins. Only one specimen was found positive for EBER, and one was found positive for multiple lytic EBV proteins. Finally, Sargsyan and colleagues employed real-time PCR to detect EBV RNA transcripts in 15 fresh-frozen MS plaques, 5 formalin-fixed paraffin embedded plaques, including 3 that tested positive for EBV in a previous study. Evidence of viral transcripts was only found in the specimens known to be positive for EBV.

How can these different results be reconciled? Diffuse EBV infection was found only in patients that had ectopic B cell follicles in the meninges. Moreover Aloisi's group argues that preserving meninges in frozen and paraffin embedded tissue section might be challenging and meninges can be lost during tissue sectioning [Aloisi et al. 2010]. They also pointed out that there are issues regarding RNA preservation: in fact, other groups did not detect EBER signal despite positive results for viral protein and viral DNA and this could indicate that RNA might have been degraded [Aloisi et al. 2010]. Finally Aloisi's group explains that other groups used RNA isolated from an entire section without performing any EBV cDNA pre-enrichment prior to PCR analysis. Whole section approaches could be less sensitive and well below the detection limit [Aloisi et al. 2010; Serafini et al. 2010]. It is unlikely that these results are false negative or false positive: Aloisi's tissue sections were selected from patients with prominent B cells infiltration and high levels of inflammation (in the case of the two acute MS cases). On the other hand, the articles with disparities are looking at less well-selected tissues that are not enriched in B cells infiltrations or ectopic follicles structures. Future studies should focus on the prevalence of B cells infiltration and ectopic follicles by screening plaques from different patients at different disease stages to confirm if EBV infection is a common feature of a certain subset of patients.

EBV Infection of Cell Types other than B Cells

Inconsistent EBV detection in the CNS of MS patients indicates that EBV might be triggering disease by infecting a small subset of cells in the CNS or by another mechanism. The presence of autoreactive myelin-specific lymphocytes is not sufficient to cause MS and such cells have been isolated from healthy individuals [Tejada-Simon et al. 2000; Ota et al. 1990]. In mouse models, MS-like disease can be triggered only after a leakage of the blood brain barrier (BBB) [Brabb et al. 1997; Millward et al. 2007]. The BBB is critical for maintenance of brain homeostasis. Brain vessels are composed of a specialized type of endothelial cell that protects the brain by preventing the passage of molecules and immune cells. In MS patients, the formation of new demyelination plaques is associated with a disruption of the BBB [Correale et al. 2007]. Intriguingly, EBV has been shown to infect other types of cells like endothelial cells [Jones et al. 1995; Xiong et al. 2004]. We recently published an article demonstrating that EBV can infect human brain microvessel endothelial cells (HBMECs) that compose the endothelium of the BBB [Casiraghi et al. 2011]. Further, we showed that EBV infection of HBMECs leads to endothelial cell activation with upregulation of RANTES and ICAM-1 and increased PBMCs adhesion. We propose that reactivation of EBV infection in the endothelium of the BBB could upregulate pro-inflammatory molecules that would induce a local breach in the BBB thereby attracting and providing entry to autoreactive lymphocytes into the CNS. In an individual with an increased level of peripheral autoreactive T cells, this could lead to an initial localized entry of immune cells and the development of MS lesions and plaques. EBV reactivation only needs to occur within a small percentage of these cells. This proposed model could also explain the inconsistent detection of EBV within MS brains. Finally, this model may work in concert with other mechanisms including EBV influence on B cells or APCs. Future studies should investigate the possible role in MS of EBV infection in other cell targets; not only endothelial cells but also epithelial cells [Hutt-Fletcher 2007] and monocytes [Savard et al. 2000].

Conclusion

In conclusion, there is convincing epidemiological evidence that EBV is involved in MS but the pathogenic mechanisms remain elusive. It is conceivable that genetically susceptible individuals infected by this virus could respond differently to other infections leading to the development of an autoimmune response. Anti-B cell therapies have been recently proven to be very effective for the treatment of MS [Hauser et al. 2008], but it is possible that prolonged B cell depletion could impair immune responses to pathogens and thus it may not be the best therapeutic approach. The monoclonal antibody used in these clinical trials is rituximab and targets CD20 that is expressed on the surface of all B cells excluding plasma cells. Antibody production is not affected by this therapy and rituximab treated subjects maintain a stable antibody titer. This indicates that antibodies produced by MS patients are likely non pathogenic and B cells might contributing to disease by acting as antigen presenting cells or by producing pro-inflammatory mediators that prime and sustain an autoreactive T cell response. Previous studies focused mainly on the humoral and cellular immune response against EBV in MS patients and on the presence of EBV infection in the CNS. EBV infects and transforms B cells, so future studies should investigate the effect that EBV infection has on antigen presentation and its ability to influence polarization and cytokine expression by B cells, within the CNS or the periphery. Most notably, this should be followed in individuals that have had mononucleosis. Finally, considering that both herpesvirus reactivation and MS relapses often occur after patients are exposed to stress stimuli, future studies should also focus on the role of EBV reactivation during MS relapses in both B cells and other EBV targets like endothelial cells, at the level of the BBB, to assess if EBV could have a role in increasing BBB permeability in vivo.

References

Aloisi, F., Serafini, B., Magliozzi, R., Howell, O.W., Reynolds, R., 2010. Detection of Epstein-Barr virus and B-cell follicles in the multiple sclerosis brain: what you find depends on how and where you look. *Brain* 133, e157.

Alotaibi, S., Kennedy, J., Tellier, R., Stephens, D., Banwell, B., 2004. Epstein-Barr virus in pediatric multiple sclerosis. *JAMA* 291, 1875-1879.

Ascherio, A., Munch, M., 2000. Epstein-Barr virus and multiple sclerosis. *Epidemiology* 11, 220-224.

Ascherio, A., Munger, K.L., Lennette, E.T., Spiegelman, D., Hernan, M.A., Olek, M.J., Hankinson, S.E., Hunter, D.J., 2001. Epstein-Barr virus antibodies and risk of multiple sclerosis: a prospective study. *JAMA* 286, 3083-3088.

Banwell, B., Krupp, L., Kennedy, J., Tellier, R., Tenembaum, S., Ness, J., Belman, A., Boiko, A., Bykova, O., Waubant, E., Mah, J.K., Stoian, C., Kremenchutzky, M., Bardini, M.R., Ruggieri, M., Rensel, M., Hahn, J., Weinstock-Guttman, B., Yeh, E.A., Farrell, K., Freedman, M., Iivanainen, M., Sevon, M., Bhan, V., Dilenge, M.E., Stephens, D., Bar-Or, A., 2007. Clinical features and viral serologies in children with multiple sclerosis: a multinational observational study. *Lancet Neurol* 6, 773-781.

Brabb, T., Goldrath, A.W., von Dassow, P., Paez, A., Liggitt, H.D., Goverman, J., 1997. Triggers of autoimmune disease in a murine TCR-transgenic model for multiple sclerosis. *J Immunol* 159, 497-507.

Bray, P.F., Bloomer, L.C., Salmon, V.C., Bagley, M.H., Larsen, P.D., 1983. Epstein-Barr virus infection and antibody synthesis in patients with multiple sclerosis. *Arch Neurol* 40, 406-408.

Brennan, R.M., Burrows, J.M., Bell, M.J., Bromham, L., Csurhes, P.A., Lenarczyk, A., Sverndal, J., Klintenstedt, J., Pender, M.P., Burrows, S.R., 2010. Strains of Epstein-Barr virus infecting multiple sclerosis patients. *Mult Scler* 16, 643-651.

Burks, J.S., Johnson, K.P., Murray T.J. 2000. The history of multiple sclerosis. In: Burks JS, Johnson KP, eds. *Multiple sclerosis: diagnosis, medical management and rehabilitation.* New York: Demos, 2000:1–32.

Casiraghi, C., Dorovini-Zis, K., Horwitz, M.S., 2011. Epstein-Barr virus infection of human brain microvessel endothelial cells: a novel role in multiple sclerosis. J Neuroimmunol 230, 173-177.

Cepok, S., Zhou, D., Srivastava, R., Nessler, S., Stei, S., Bussow, K., Sommer, N., Hemmer, B., 2005. Identification of Epstein-Barr virus proteins as putative targets of the immune response in multiple sclerosis. *J Clin Invest* 115, 1352-1360.

Clanet, M., 2008. Jean-Martin Charcot. 1825 to 1893. Int MS J 15, 59-61.

Comabella, M., Montalban, X., Horga, A., Messmer, B., Kakalacheva, K., Strowig, T., Caballero, E., Munz, C., Lunemann, J., 2010. Antiviral immune response in patients with multiple sclerosis and healthy siblings. Mult Scler 16, 355-358.

Correale, J., Villa, A., 2007. The blood-brain-barrier in multiple sclerosis: functional roles and therapeutic targeting. *Autoimmunity* 40, 148-160.

Craig, J.C., Haire, M., Millar, J.H., Fraser, K.B., Merrett, J.D., 1983. Immunological control of Epstein-Barr virus-transformed lymphocytes in multiple sclerosis. *Clin Immunol Immunopathol* 29, 86-93.

Craig, J.C., Hawkins, S.A., Swallow, M.W., Lyttle, J.A., Patterson, V.H., Merrett, J.D., Haire, M., 1985. Subsets of T lymphocytes in relation to T lymphocyte function in multiple sclerosis. *Clin Exp Immunol 61*, 548-555.

Craig, J.C., Haire, M., Merrett, J.D., 1988. T-cell-mediated suppression of Epstein-Barr virus-induced B lymphocyte activation in multiple sclerosis. *Clin Immunol Immunopathol* 48, 253-260.

DeLorenze, G.N., Munger, K.L., Lennette, E.T., Orentreich, N., Vogelman, J.H., Ascherio, A., 2006. Epstein-Barr virus and multiple sclerosis: evidence of association from a prospective study with long-term follow-up. *Arch Neurol* 63, 839-844.

Esposito, M., Venkatesh, V., Otvos, L., Weng, Z., Vajda, S., Banki, K., Perl, A., 1999. Human transaldolase and cross-reactive viral epitopes identified by autoantibodies of multiple sclerosis patients. *J Immunol* 163, 4027-4032.

Farrell, R.A., Antony, D., Wall, G.R., Clark, D.A., Fisniku, L., Swanton, J., Khaleeli, Z., Schmierer, K., Miller, D.H., Giovannoni, G., 2009. Humoral immune response to EBV in multiple sclerosis is associated with disease activity on MRI. *Neurology* 73, 32-38.

Franciotta, D., Di Stefano, A.L., Jarius, S., Zardini, E., Tavazzi, E., Ballerini, C., Marchioni, E., Bergamaschi, R., Ceroni, M., 2010. Cerebrospinal BAFF and Epstein-Barr virus-specific oligoclonal bands in multiple sclerosis and other inflammatory demyelinating neurological diseases. *J Neuroimmunol* 230, 160-163.

Fraser, K.B., Haire, M., Millar, J.H., McCrea, S., 1979. Increased tendency to spontaneous in-vitro lymphocyte transformation in clinically active multiple sclerosis. *Lancet* 2, 175-176.

Gronen, F., Ruprecht, K., Weissbrich, B., Klinker, E., Kroner, A., Hofstetter, H.H., Rieckmann, P., 2006. Frequency analysis of HLA-B7-restricted Epstein-Barr virus-specific cytotoxic T lymphocytes in patients with multiple sclerosis and healthy controls. *J Neuroimmunol* 180, 185-192.

Handel, A.E., Williamson, A.J., Disanto, G., Handunnetthi, L., Giovannoni, G., Ramagopalan, S.V., 2009. An updated meta-analysis of risk of multiple sclerosis following infectious mononucleosis. *PLoS One* 5(9) e12496.

Hauser, S.L., Waubant, E., Arnold, D.L., Vollmer, T., Antel, J., Fox, R.J., Bar-Or, A., Panzara, M., Sarkar, N., Agarwal, S., Langer-Gould, A., Smith, C.H., 2008. B-cell depletion with rituximab in relapsing-remitting multiple sclerosis. *N Engl J Med* 358, 676-688.

Hilton, D.A., Love, S., Fletcher, A., Pringle, J.H., 1994. Absence of Epstein-Barr virus RNA in multiple sclerosis as assessed by in situ hybridisation. *J Neurol Neurosurg Psychiatry* 57, 975-976.

Hollsberg, P., Hansen, H.J., Haahr, S., 2003. Altered CD8+ T cell responses to selected Epstein-Barr virus immunodominant epitopes in patients with multiple sclerosis. *Clin Exp Immunol* 132, 137-143.

Holmoy, T., Kvale, E.O., Vartdal, F., 2004. Cerebrospinal fluid CD4+ T cells from a multiple sclerosis patient cross-recognize Epstein-Barr virus and myelin basic protein. *J Neurovirol* 10, 278-283.

Hutt-Fletcher, L.M., 2007. Epstein-Barr virus entry. *J Virol* 81, 7825-7832.

Jafari, N., van Nierop, G.P., Verjans, G.M., Osterhaus, A.D., Middeldorp, J.M., Hintzen, R.Q., 2010. No evidence for intrathecal IgG synthesis to Epstein Barr virus nuclear antigen-1 in multiple sclerosis. *J Clin Virol* 49, 26-31.

Jaquiery, E., Jilek, S., Schluep, M., Meylan, P., Lysandropoulos, A., Pantaleo, G., Du Pasquier, R.A., 2010a. Intrathecal immune responses to EBV in early MS. *Eur J Immunol* 40, 878-887.

Jaquiery, E., Jilek, S., Schluep, M., Le Goff, G., Garcia, M., Pantaleo, G., Du Pasquier, R.A., 2010b. Cytokine mRNA profile of Epstein-Barr virus-stimulated highly differentiated T cells in multiple sclerosis: a pilot study. *J Neuroimmunol 225*, 167-170.

Jilek, S., Schluep, M., Meylan, P., Vingerhoets, F., Guignard, L., Monney, A., Kleeberg, J., Le Goff, G., Pantaleo, G., Du Pasquier, R.A., 2008. Strong EBV-specific CD8+ T-cell response in patients with early multiple sclerosis. *Brain* 131, 1712-1721.

Jones, K., Rivera, C., Sgadari, C., Franklin, J., Max, E.E., Bhatia, K., Tosato, G., 1995. Infection of human endothelial cells with Epstein-Barr virus. *J Exp Med* 182, 1213-1221.

Kieff, E., Rickinson, A.B.: *Epstein-Barr Virus and its replication.* In *Fields Virology*. 5th edition. Edited by Fields BN, Knipe DM, Howley PM. Lippincott-Williams & Wilkins Publishers: Philadelphia; 2007:2603-2654.

Lang, H.L., Jacobsen, H., Ikemizu, S., Andersson, C., Harlos, K., Madsen, L., Hjorth, P., Sondergaard, L., Svejgaard, A., Wucherpfennig, K., Stuart, D.I., Bell, J.I., Jones, E.Y., Fugger, L., 2002. A functional and structural basis for TCR cross-reactivity in multiple sclerosis. *Nat Immunol* 3, 940-943.

Levin, L.I., Munger, K.L., Rubertone, M.V., Peck, C.A., Lennette, E.T., Spiegelman, D., Ascherio, A., 2005. Temporal relationship between elevation of epstein-barr virus antibody titers and initial onset of neurological symptoms in multiple sclerosis. *JAMA* 293, 2496-2500.

Levin, L.I., Munger, K.L., O'Reilly, E.J., Falk, K.I., Ascherio, A., 2010. Primary infection with the Epstein-Barr virus and risk of multiple sclerosis. *Ann Neurol* 67, 824-830.

Lindsey, J.W., Patel, S., Zou, J., 2008. Epstein-Barr virus genotypes in multiple sclerosis. *Acta Neurol Scand* 117, 141-144.

Lindsey, J.W., Hatfield, L.M., Crawford, M.P., Patel, S., 2009. Quantitative PCR for Epstein-Barr virus DNA and RNA in multiple sclerosis. *Mult Scler* 15, 153-158.

Lindsey, J.W., Hatfield, L.M., 2010. Epstein-Barr virus and multiple sclerosis: cellular immune response and cross-reactivity. *J Neuroimmunol* 229, 238-242.

Lunemann, J.D., Edwards, N., Muraro, P.A., Hayashi, S., Cohen, J.I., Munz, C., Martin, R., 2006. Increased frequency and broadened specificity of latent EBV nuclear antigen-1-specific T cells in multiple sclerosis. *Brain* 129, 1493-1506.

Lunemann, J.D., Huppke, P., Roberts, S., Bruck, W., Gartner, J., Munz, C., 2008a. Broadened and elevated humoral immune response to EBNA1 in pediatric multiple sclerosis. *Neurology* 71, 1033-1035.

Lunemann, J.D., Jelcic, I., Roberts, S., Lutterotti, A., Tackenberg, B., Martin, R., Munz, C., 2008b. EBNA1-specific T cells from patients with multiple sclerosis cross react with myelin antigens and co-produce IFN-gamma and IL-2. *J Exp Med* 205, 1763-1773.

Lunemann, J.D., Tintore, M., Messmer, B., Strowig, T., Rovira, A., Perkal, H., Caballero, E., Munz, C., Montalban, X., Comabella, M., 2010. Elevated Epstein-Barr virus-encoded nuclear antigen-1 immune responses predict conversion to multiple sclerosis. *Ann Neurol* 67, 159-169.

Martin, R., Voskuhl, R., Flerlage, M., McFarlin, D.E., McFarland, H.F., 1993. Myelin basic protein-specific T-cell responses in identical twins discordant or concordant for multiple sclerosis. *Ann Neurol* 34, 524-535.

Massa, J., Munger, K.L., O'Reilly, E.J., Falk, K.I., Ascherio, A., 2007. Plasma titers of antibodies against Epstein-Barr virus BZLF1 and risk of multiple sclerosis. *Neuroepidemiology* 28, 214-215.

Millward, J.M., Caruso, M., Campbell, I.L., Gauldie, J., Owens, T., 2007. IFN-gamma-induced chemokines synergize with pertussis toxin to promote T cell entry to the central nervous system. *J Immunol* 178, 8175-8182.

Morre, S.A., van Beek, J., De Groot, C.J., Killestein, J., Meijer, C.J., Polman, C.H., van der Valk, P., Middeldorp, J.M., van Den Brule, A.J., 2001. Is Epstein-Barr virus present in the CNS of patients with MS? *Neurology* 56, 692.

Myhr, K.M., Riise, T., Barrett-Connor, E., Myrmel, H., Vedeler, C., Gronning, M., Kalvenes, M.B., Nyland, H., 1998. Altered antibody pattern to Epstein-Barr virus but not to other herpesviruses in multiple sclerosis: a population based case-control study from western Norway. *J Neurol Neurosurg Psychiatry* 64, 539-542.

Nielsen, T.R., Rostgaard, K., Askling, J., Steffensen, R., Oturai, A., Jersild, C., Koch-Henriksen, N., Sorensen, P.S., Hjalgrim, H., 2009. Effects of infectious mononucleosis and HLA-DRB1*15 in multiple sclerosis. *Mult Scler* 15, 431-436.

Nociti, V., Frisullo, G., Marti, A., Luigetti, M., Iorio, R., Patanella, A.K., Bianco, A., Tonali, P.A., Grillo, R.L., Sabatelli, M., Batocchi, A.P., 2010. Epstein-Barr virus antibodies in serum and cerebrospinal fluid from multiple sclerosis, chronic inflammatory demyelinating polyradiculoneuropathy and amyotrophic lateral sclerosis. *J Neuroimmunol* 225, 149-152.

Opsahl, M.L., Kennedy, P.G., 2007. An attempt to investigate the presence of Epstein Barr virus in multiple sclerosis and normal control brain tissue. *J Neurol* 254, 425-430.

Ota, K., Matsui, M., Milford, E.L., Mackin, G.A., Weiner, H.L., Hafler, D.A., 1990. T-cell recognition of an immunodominant myelin basic protein epitope in multiple sclerosis. *Nature* 346, 183-187.

Peferoen, L.A., Lamers, F., Lodder, L.N., Gerritsen, W.H., Huitinga, I., Melief, J., Giovannoni, G., Meier, U., Hintzen, R.Q., Verjans, G.M., van Nierop, G.P., Vos, W., Peferoen-Baert, R.M., Middeldorp, J.M., van der Valk, P., Amor, S., 2010. Epstein Barr virus is not a characteristic feature in the central nervous system in established multiple sclerosis. *Brain* 133, e137.

Pender, M.P., Csurhes, P.A., Lenarczyk, A., Pfluger, C.M., Burrows, S.R., 2009. Decreased T cell reactivity to Epstein-Barr virus infected lymphoblastoid cell lines in multiple sclerosis. *J Neurol Neurosurg Psychiatry* 80, 498-505.

Pohl, D., Krone, B., Rostasy, K., Kahler, E., Brunner, E., Lehnert, M., Wagner, H.J., Gartner, J., Hanefeld, F., 2006. High seroprevalence of Epstein-Barr virus in children with multiple sclerosis. *Neurology* 67, 2063-2065.

Pohl, D., Rostasy, K., Jacobi, C., Lange, P., Nau, R., Krone, B., Hanefeld, F., 2009. Intrathecal antibody production against Epstein-Barr and other neurotropic viruses in pediatric and adult onset multiple sclerosis. *J Neurol* 257, 212-216.

Ramagopalan, S.V., Valdar, W., Dyment, D.A., DeLuca, G.C., Yee, I.M., Giovannoni, G., Ebers, G.C., Sadovnick, A.D., 2009. Association of infectious mononucleosis with multiple sclerosis. A population-based study. *Neuroepidemiology* 32, 257-262.

Rand, K.H., Houck, H., Denslow, N.D., Heilman, K.M., 1998. Molecular approach to find target(s) for oligoclonal bands in multiple sclerosis. *J Neurol Neurosurg Psychiatry* 65, 48-55.

Rand, K.H., Houck, H., Denslow, N.D., Heilman, K.M., 2000. Epstein-Barr virus nuclear antigen-1 (EBNA-1) associated oligoclonal bands in patients with multiple sclerosis. *J Neurol Sci* 173, 32-39.

Sargsyan, S.A., Shearer, A.J., Ritchie, A.M., Burgoon, M.P., Anderson, S., Hemmer, B., Stadelmann, C., Gattenlohner, S., Owens, G.P., Gilden, D., Bennett, J.L., 2010. Absence of Epstein-Barr virus in the brain and CSF of patients with multiple sclerosis. *Neurology* 74, 1127-1135.

Savard, M., Belanger, C., Tardif, M., Gourde, P., Flamand, L., Gosselin, J., 2000. Infection of primary human monocytes by Epstein-Barr virus. *J Virol* 74, 2612-2619.

Serafini, B., Rosicarelli, B., Franciotta, D., Magliozzi, R., Reynolds, R., Cinque, P., Andreoni, L., Trivedi, P., Salvetti, M., Faggioni, A., Aloisi, F., 2007. Dysregulated Epstein-Barr virus infection in the multiple sclerosis brain. *J Exp Med* 204, 2899-2912.

Serafini, B., Severa, M., Columba-Cabezas, S., Rosicarelli, B., Veroni, C., Chiappetta, G., Magliozzi, R., Reynolds, R., Coccia, E.M., Aloisi, F., 2010. Epstein-Barr virus latent infection and BAFF expression in B cells in the multiple sclerosis brain: implications for viral persistence and intrathecal B-cell activation. J *Neuropathol Exp Neurol* 69, 677-693.

Simon, K.C., Yang, X., Munger, K.L., Ascherio, A., 2010. *EBNA1 and LMP1 variants in multiple sclerosis cases and controls.* Acta Neurol Scand. In press

Sospedra, M., Martin, R., 2005. Immunology of multiple sclerosis. *Annu Rev Immunol* 23, 683-747.

Sumaya, C.V., Myers, L.W., Ellison, G.W., 1980. Epstein-Barr virus antibodies in multiple sclerosis. *Arch Neurol* 37, 94-96.

Sundstrom, P., Juto, P., Wadell, G., Hallmans, G., Svenningsson, A., Nystrom, L., Dillner, J., Forsgren, L., 2004. An altered immune response to Epstein-Barr virus in multiple sclerosis: a prospective study. *Neurology* 62, 2277-2282.

Tejada-Simon, M.V., Zang, Y.C., Yang, D., Hong, J., Li, S., Singh, R.A., Van den Berg-Loonen, E., Killian, J.M., Rivera, V.M., Zhang, J.Z., 2000. Aberrant T cell responses to myelin antigens during clinical exacerbation in patients with multiple sclerosis. *Int Immunol* 12, 1641-1650.

Vaughan, J.H., Riise, T., Rhodes, G.H., Nguyen, M.D., Barrett-Connor, E., Nyland, H., 1996. An Epstein Barr virus-related cross reactive autoimmune response in multiple sclerosis in Norway. *J Neuroimmunol* 69, 95-102.

Wagner, H.J., Munger, K.L., Ascherio, A., 2004. Plasma viral load of Epstein-Barr virus and risk of multiple sclerosis. *Eur J Neurol* 11, 833-834.

Wandinger, K., Jabs, W., Siekhaus, A., Bubel, S., Trillenberg, P., Wagner, H., Wessel, K., Kirchner, H., Hennig, H., 2000. Association between clinical disease activity and Epstein-Barr virus reactivation in MS. *Neurology* 55, 178-184.

Warner, H.B., Carp, R.I., 1981. Multiple sclerosis and Epstein-Barr virus. *Lancet* 2, 1290.

Warner, H.B., Carp, R.I., 1988. Multiple sclerosis etiology--an Epstein-Barr virus hypothesis. *Med Hypotheses* 25, 93-97.

Willis, S.N., Stadelmann, C., Rodig, S.J., Caron, T., Gattenloehner, S., Mallozzi, S.S., Roughan, J.E., Almendinger, S.E., Blewett, M.M., Bruck, W., Hafler, D.A., O'Connor, K.C., 2009. Epstein-Barr virus infection is not a characteristic feature of multiple sclerosis brain. *Brain* 132, 3318-3328.

Wucherpfennig, K.W., Strominger, J.L., 1995. Molecular mimicry in T cell-mediated autoimmunity: viral peptides activate human T cell clones specific for myelin basic protein. *Cell* 80, 695-705.

Xiong, A., Clarke-Katzenberg, R.H., Valenzuela, G., Izumi, K.M., Millan, M.T., 2004. Epstein-Barr virus latent membrane protein 1 activates nuclear factor-kappa B in human endothelial cells and inhibits apoptosis. *Transplantation 78*, 41-49.

Zivadinov, R., Zorzon, M., Weinstock-Guttman, B., Serafin, M., Bosco, A., Bratina, A., Maggiore, C., Grop, A., Tommasi, M.A., Srinivasaraghavan, B., Ramanathan, M., 2009. Epstein-Barr virus is associated with grey matter atrophy in multiple sclerosis. *J Neurol Neurosurg Psychiatry* 80, 620-625.

In: Multiple Sclerosis
Editor: E. Scholz and C. Müller, pp. 97-112
ISBN 978-1-61324-848-5

Chapter V

Actual Relation between Multiple Sclerosis and Epstein-Barr Virus

Olivia Santiago[a]***, Antonio Sorlozano***[a]***, Maria José Soto***[a]***,***
Enrique Villegas[a]***, Jose Gutierrez***[a,b,*]
[a]Department of Microbiology, School of Medicine, University of Granada, Spain
[b]Service of Microbiology, University Hospital "Virgen de las Nieves", Granada, Spain

Abstract

Multiple sclerosis is a demyelinating disease that affects the central nervous system and one of the most common causes of neurologic disability in young adults. Although its pathogenesis is not clear, it seems to have an immune basis in genetically-sensitive persons. Some factors, most of them still unknown, may trigger the activation of the immune system to produce inflammatory damages that may include demyelination, axonal damages and oligodendrocyte loss, followed by structural repair, post-inflammatory gliosis and neurodegeneration.

Over the past 50 years, a great number of work groups have researched the possible participation of infectious agents in multiple sclerosis, and a significant number of microorganisms have been proposed as possible candidates in the pathogenesis of this inflammatory and demyelinating process. Amongst the numerous candidate microorganisms, many publications have linked viruses from the *Herpesviridae* family, especially, the Epstein-Barr virus, to the disease.

Several hypotheses have been proposed in an attempt to explain the role of this virus. That is the case of the molecular mimetic hypothesis, infection of autoimmune B-cells, superantigen and αB-crystallin protein, or the hygiene hypothesis. Nonetheless, the diversity of results obtained shows the need for an analytic summary of the findings of all the scientific literature available in order to integrate them and establish whether there is any real evidence of an association between infection and disease, defining a possible

[*] Corresponding author: Jose Gutierrez. Department of Microbiology, School of Medicine, Avd de Madrid, 11, E-18012 Granada, Spain. Tel. 34-958020465; Fax: 34-958246119; E-mail: josegf@ugr.es

theoretical framework on the scientific knowledge available on the issue that may subsequently be useful in clinical practice and health care.

Possible Relationship between Infection by Epstein-Barr Virus (EBV) and Multiple Sclerosis (MS)

Various studies have posed several hypotheses involving different microorganisms in the pathogenesis of multiple sclerosis (MS). The hygiene hypothesis, for instance, states that childhood exposure to the infectious agent is associated with a reduced risk of MS, but a later infection by the same agent increases such risk [1]. However, other authors believe this hypothesis fails to explain cases without any history of contact with said infectious agents [2]. On the other hand, Kurtzke's or prevalence hypothesis, based on an epidemiology study carried out on the Faroe Islands, states that MS may be caused by a pathogen that is more common in regions with high prevalence of the disease [3].

In any case, several studies have related over 14 infectious agents with the pathogenesis of MS [4,5]. The *Herpesviridae* family was the most studied, and ample evidence relating Epstein-Barr virus (EBV) infection with MS was provided.

The first association between the epidemiology of MS and EBV infection was established in 1981 [6], and this association has since then been widely studied, an interest maybe due to the fact, as some authors insist, that MS epidemiology is extremely parallel to that of infectious mononucleosis (IM) [7,8].

It has already been stated that in Northern European countries (Denmark, for example), contact of a third of all EBV-infected cases takes place during puberty or adulthood, while in Southern European countries infection occurs mainly during the early years of life. IM appearing during childhood is generally subclinical and more frequent in low socio-economic status societies. Several authors blame it on the low levels of hygiene and health care, which promote contact with the virus at an early age. IM also does appear at a later age, although with generally richer symptoms, and is more frequent in high socio-economic status societies, in which pathogen contact is delayed due to improved hygiene and sanitary conditions. Similar to the IM situation described above, MS is more prevalent in geographic areas with high socio-economic status [8].

A study on the Norwegian population observed that MS patients' birth dates showed proximity, with ages ranging between 13 and 20. It was also noted that they had lived in close areas and that they shared similar risk factors, such as EBV infection, which was determined to be the main factor explaining this accumulation of cases [9].

Other factors that have been related to MS and EBV infection are: vitamin D deficit and exposure to the sun. Grant's [10] study showed that 1,25-dihydroxi-vitamin D metabolite induces the production of cathelicidin (LL-37), a peptide with antimicrobial activity which prevents both viral and bacterial infections.This may partly explain the fact that infections are more frequent during cold seasons, when vitamin D production, which is dependent upon UV radiation, is lower.It has been proven in EBV cases that diseases such as IM have incidence peaks in winter [11].

Based on this and other epidemiological coincidences between both diseases, many studies have analyzed the relative risk of developing MS in individuals who have suffered IM [4,12-19]. Some of these studies have led us to believe that later EBV infection may be an aetiological factor in the development of MS.

Given that there may be a relationship between EBV infection and MS, several pathogenic hypotheses have been posed in the attempt to explain the contribution of the virus to this disease.

Molecular Mimicry Hypothesis

This is currently the prevailing hypothesis. It is based on the homology between the virus proteins and myelin proteins [20-25]. According to this hypothesis, T- and B-cells, which may become active against the body's own antigens, may also become active against epitopes of some infectious agents, crossing the hematoencephalic barrier (HEB) and causing an inflammatory reaction in the central nervous system (CNS) [7].

T-cell response may initiate and sustain MS autoimmunity, since certain specific CD4+ T-cells exist against the basic myelin protein and also recognize EBV epitopes [25]. These cells are increased in MS patients and they are specific against the virus nuclear protein, EBNA1, such that myelin-specific auto-antigen cross-recognition may occur [23,26,27]. Lang *et al.* [22] proved that one of the clones of CD4+ T-cells presenting cross-reaction in MS patients recognizes the myelin basic protein peptide through the HLA DRB1*1501 molecule, and the virus through HLA DRB5*0101, both of which happen to be the two HLA molecules most associated with MS.

Cytotoxic CD8+ T-cells, which recognize the presence of epitopes through the HLA-B7 molecule, have also been found to be increased in MS patients, especially in remitting-recurrent cases [28]. Nevertheless, other authors have determined that EBV epitope targets for CD8+ T-cells are not different between MS patients and healthy controls [26].

According to the molecular mimicry hypothesis, MS may combine a genetic predisposition with an infectious factor, thus maintaining auto-reactive T-cells which may result in the disease [23,29].

EBV-infected Autoimmune B-cells Hypothesis

Pender [30] also proposed a hypothesis to explain the role of EBV in the development of the disease, in which MS may be produced through the accumulation of infected auto-reactive B-cells in the CNS. This hypothesis would involve the virus's immortalization capacity and its molecular mimicry capacity, in addition to CD4+ T-cells being able to recognize auto-antigens. The pathogenic mechanism would be as follows:

- EBV would infect a great number of B-cells and auto-reactive B-cells during primary infection.
- These B-cells would multiply regardless of T-cell activation signals because EBV infection-acquired LMP1 proteins, homologous to the CD40 molecule, render them

capable of this, and rescue B-cells from apoptosis, transform their morphology, reduce the normal differentiation signal response and facilitate their proliferation [31-33]. With BCR functional homology, in absence of a competent BCR that may translate signals and an antigen to activate them [33], these cells may be maintained through LMP2A. Other viral genes [34] may also influence this proliferation, transformation and immortalization of B-cells.

- Thus, latent infected memory B-cells would continue their circulation in the blood as a result of the EBV infection.
- These infected B-cells would normally be eliminated by specific CD8+ T-cells, but if there is a genetic defect in the mechanism, this elimination would be impossible.
- In MS, these antigen-specific activated autoimmune B-cells may cross the HEB and lodge in the CNS, where they would persist, continuously dodging apoptosis through the expression of certain genes, such as BHRF1 [35,36], LMP1 [37] and EBNA1 [38].
- Infected B-cells in the CNS may also act as antigen presenter cells for T-cells. When CD4+ T-cells recognizing CNS antigens are activated in lymphoid organs through cross-reaction with EBV antigens, they migrate to the CNS and lodge in the target organ presenting the auto-antigen with which they react. These cells are normally eliminated in the target organ through induced apoptosis, but if they react with infected auto-reactive B-cells accumulated in the organ, they receive the survival signal that inhibits their apoptosis.
- Surviving CD4+ T-cells activate other mature B-cells to produce antibodies which react with the target organ and damage the CNS. These autoimmune T-cells proliferate and produce cytokines that recruit other inflammatory cells; as a result, damage in the myelin occurs. This response may trigger the liberation of auto-antigens and promote the activation of other T and B-cells, and an immune response against other antigens.
- In addition, independent of the whole process, production of new viral particles with infectious capacity may be under way, since the differentiation of latent infected memory B-cells to plasma cells may provoke the entry of the virus in the lytic cycle [33]. Thus, the autoimmune process produces a vicious circle where EBV-infected B-cells promote autoimmunity and CNS viral infection [30].

The analysis of the results found in the bibliography on the possible association between EBV and MS may allow us to observe findings that indicate this hypothesis may be contrasted. It is clear that intrathecal synthesis of antibodies is characteristic of MS and that clonally expanded B-cells contribute to increased IgG in the CSF [39]; monoclonal IgG is present in MS as oligoclonal bands (OB) [40,41] and the majority are directed against infectious agents. Thus, this intense humoral response posed against EBV may influence MS pathogenesis, since it is a long-term response and remains for several years after infection [42-44].

Infected B- and plasma cell infiltration has also been observed in the active lesions of the disease, with formation of ectopic B-cell follicles in the meninges, the main place of viral persistence [45]. These B-cell follicles show germinal centre characteristics, where these cells may proliferate, differentiate and mature, expressing EBERs, EBNA2 and LMP1 [45]. The presence of these B-cells in the brain contributes to MS pathogenesis since, in addition to acting as antigen presenter cells, they may produce antibodies specific against myelin antigens [24,42,46]. Other authors have however not been able to reproduce these results [47,48].

Superantigen Hypothesis

The spontaneous *in vitro* transformation of infected B-cells results, in addition to new EBV particles, in endogenous retroviruses [49], which may transcribe a gene codifying a capsule protein with possible activity as superantigen [8,50]. Specifically, EBV activates HERV-K18 transcription in B-cells, which could contribute to the death of oligodendrocytes and to MS pathogenesis. The action of EBV in this pathogenetic mechanism would be indirect [8].

EBV also has the capacity to induce the expression of αB-crystallin protein in the surface of B-cells. This protein is absent in human lymphoid tissue, so that the immune system does not tolerate it, which could trigger CD4+ T-cells appearance and also the appearance of the response against it. This protein is identified as the greatest auto-antigen abnormally expressed in brain oligodendrocytes in MS patients and it is highly expressed in early lesions of the disease. It has been suggested that it is an immunodominant myelin antigen for T-cells in the CNS of persons affected by MS [51-54].

Hygiene Hypothesis

Lastly, the hygiene hypothesis [1,55] may explain the increase in the incidence of MS in the developed world. It is based on the observation of an increase in the prevalence of autoimmune diseases in countries with notable reduction of infections by classic or prevalent pathogens and it explains that the interaction of humans with prevalent pathogens prevents the appearance of autoimmune diseases [56].

Thus, protection against autoimmune diseases such as MS may be conferred by persistent effects in the immune response during a microbial or parasitic infection during childhood, something which favours the correct development of the immune system, since it has a great regulatory mesh that is genetically determined but which matures according to the nature of the person, the calendar of infections and other changes suffered during childhood [57]. Childhood infections stimulate the production of regulating cells, such as T-lymphocytes, and they prevent the collateral damage to tissues associated to prolonged inflammatory responses [58]. The absence of infections during childhood may alter the process and favour the development of autoimmune diseases due to the poor action of regulating T-cells [56].

It has been proven that regulating T-cells in MS patients present defects in their suppressing capacity [59], which may be a key element in the disease pathogenesis. Differences have also been spotted in the suppressing capacity of cytokine production of regulating T-cells, results which indicate differences in the function of modulating cells that may contribute to the disease pathogenesis.

Table 1. Results of meta-analysis of the experimental works have studied the possible association between EBV and MS [92]

Determination	*OR*	95% CI	*P* value	X^2_{exp}	I^2 Higgins
Anti-VCA IgG	5.5	3.37-8.81	*<0.0001*	19.74, 12 df, *p=0.072*	39.2%
Anti-EBNA complex IgG	5.4	2.94-9.76	*<0.0001*	0.85, 4 df, *p= 0.932*	0%
Anti-EBNA1 IgG	12.1	3.13-46.89	*<0.0001*	65.76, 6 df, *p<0.0001*	90.9%
Anti-EA IgG	1.3	0.68-2.35	*0.457*	20.30, 5 df, *p=0.001*	75.4%
HA	1.9	1.56-2.36	*<0.0001*	2.57, 3 df, *p=0.463*	0%
DNA (BL)	1.8	0.99-3.36	*0.051*	10.34, 5 df, *p=0.066*	51.6%
DNA (CSF/BT)	0.9	0.38-2.01	*0.768*	3.26, 6 df, *p=0.776*	0%

HA: heterophile antibodies; BL: blood; CSF: cerebrospinal fluid; BT: brain tissue; df: degrees of freedom.

Following the analysis above, we believe it is currently necessary to summarize the results of what scientific literature is available in order to integrate them and establish whether or not statistically significant evidence exists associating EBV infection and MS, defining a possible theoretical framework of the scientific knowledge available on the issue that may subsequently be useful in the clinical and health care practice.

Statistical Analysis of Experimental Studies Showing Association between EBV Infection and MS

The web access bibliography database MEDLINE was used to find the studies and the open search was established using "Epstein-Barr virus" or "EBV" or "human herpesvirus 4" or "HHV-4" or "infectious mononucleosis" and "multiple sclerosis" as key words. The search was limited to works published in English and Spanish up to January 2009; case and control studies, cases and controls embedded in a cohort and prospective cohort studies were accepted. The requirements assessed were the inclusion of MS patients at any moment of the study and the fact that its objective was the direct or indirect search for EBV infection markers, trying to establish a possible association of the infection with the disease. Excluded were revisions, non-original articles, animal studies and those which did not assess EBV infection as risk factor for the disease; also excluded were those not available on the Web and not found by any other means, because they were not available in libraries.

Strictly following and assessing the abovementioned inclusion and exclusion criteria, 73 articles were finally selected out of 251 publications.

A total of 35 studies that only offered a percentage or a risk measurement, were discarded because they did not offer absolute results.

The search in their bibliography yielded no additional articles, so the systematic review of the bibliography yielded a total number of articles selected of 38 studies [13-17,20,60-91].

Upon selecting the works to be studied, data were extracted through a systematic procedure that required the filling in of a form created earlier. The data obtained were included in a meta-analysis, a set of statistical techniques that allows the combination of the results of independent studies on the same issue. Said work was published [92] and we can extract its most important conclusions (table 1).

The global estimate of the *OR* of individual results obtained from studies that determined the presence of anti-VCA IgG in serum [61,64-66,76,80,81,84,86-88,91] and CSF [20] led us to conclude that significant association exists between the microorganism and the disease (*OR*=5.5; CI 95%=3.37-8.81; $p<0.0001$).

The antibody titre in MS patients was significantly higher than in control subjects [20,64,66,80,84,86,87,91,93,94] in all of the studies with quantitative determination of anti-VCA IgG, and which, due to the methodology, were not included in the meta-analysis. Considering that the anti-VCA IgG antibody is a past infection marker, we may state that EBV past infection is a prerequisite for developing the disease, such that the virus may require a latency period after which the risk of having MS increases. This same hypothetical pattern has been found in other diseases associated with this virus, such as Burkitt's lymphoma [95], nasopharyngeal carcinoma [96], Hodgkin's lymphoma [97], chronic lymphocytic leukaemia [98], systemic lupus erythematosus [99,100], rheumatoid arthritis [84] and other immunodeficiency states [101,102].

The global *OR* in studies that analyzed the anti-EBNA complex IgG antibody in serum [61,64,76,82,84] indicates the existence of significant relationship between EBV exposure and MS development (*OR*=5.4; CI 95%=2.94-9.76; $p<0.0001$). The presence of these antibodies would not indicate recent, but latent infection [103] and thus we may say that their detection is related to a possible involvement of the virus in the initial pathogenesis of the disease.

A global *OR* of 12.1 was obtained from studies evaluating the anti-EBNA1 IgG antibody in CSF [20] and in serum [13,65,78,80,88,90], thus indicating statistically significant association between virus exposure and MS (CI 95%=3.13-46.89; $p<0.0001$). Antibody titres were significantly higher in cases than in controls [24,64,65,80,93,104,105] in all the studies with anti-EBNA1 IgG quantitative determination, as is the case of the anti-VCA IgG antibody. In the work by Ascherio *et al.* [64] on serum samples collected before the initial symptoms, scientists found a significant increase in the titre of anti-EBV antigen antibodies expressed during the latency phase (EBNA1 and EBNA2) and the replication phase of the virus (EA). A similar study by Levin *et al.* [105] also found a significant increase of anti-EBNA and EBNA1 complex IgG titres in the serum of subjects who had not yet developed the first symptoms of the disease. DeLorenze *et al.* [93] obtained results similar to the above with high titres of anti-EBNA1 antibodies up to 20 years before the initial symptoms, which remained constant in time. Whatever causes the elevation of these antibodies before the clinical development of MS is unknown, but it is thought to be an early manifestation of a preclinical stage of the disease, which would indicate that the increase of the antibodies' response to EBV is not a consequence of MS, but an early event in the pathogenesis later resulting in demyelination and in the clinical disease so that, in this case, a past EBV infection remains a prerequisite to developing MS.

Evidently, these findings are themselves related to the age at which the disease appeared. The study by DeLorenze *et al.* [93] showed that patients who had developed the disease in later years had anti-EBNA1 IgG antibodies that could be detected before the first symptoms of MS appeared; however, this response pattern could not be applied to people who developed the disease at an earlier time. Levin *et al.* [105] found that patients who developed MS after the age of 25 first showed an increase in the titres of anti-EBNA and EBNA-1 complex antibodies which did not appear at their early ages.

As for studies that determined anti-EA IgG [61,67,76,78,80,90] the meta-analysis discarded the possibility of any relationship between exposure to the virus and MS (OR=1.3; CI 95%=0.68-2.35; $p=0.457$). Positivity of this antibody indicates primary infection or reactivation of the virus. We may state that the presence of this antibody was not associated with the disease probably because, as we already said, EBV infection may be involved in the initial stages of MS development such that the antibody may already be undetectable by the time the disease is diagnosed.

Studies with quantitative determination of anti-EA IgG [64,103,104] also found significantly higher titres in patients versus controls, except in the DeLorenze *et al.* study [93].

The studies on heterophile antibodies (HA) [14-17] also showed a global *OR* that indicated significant association between virus exposure and MS (OR=1.9; CI 95%=1.56-2.36; $p<0.0001$).

The meta-analysis found no significant association between virus exposure and MS in the six studies that analyzed the presence of DNA in serum, two in plasma [72,89] and four in mononuclear peripheral blood cells (MPBC) [62,69,71,85], although there were signs of significance (OR=1.8; CI 95%=0.99-3.36; $p=0.051$). The presence of EBV DNA in MS patients' MPBC would only indicate that these patients were infected at some point in time and, therefore, it is possible that the virus was involved in initiating the disease pathogenesis. This further means that some authors verified the presence of the virus DNA before the first symptoms of the disease [89].

The rest of studies analyzing the presence of EBV DNA were carried out on CSF [63,68,74,75,77] and on brain tissue [77,83]. The determination of the global OR indicates that there was no significant association between virus exposure and the disease (OR=0.9; CI 95%=0.38-2.01; $p=0.768$).

Relationship between the Detection of Antibodies, Individual Genetic Factors and Multiple Sclerosis

There are studies which, in addition to determining antibodies, include the study of genetic factors associated with MS since environmental exposure to EBV alone is not, in itself, enough to explain why only some persons develop the disease. In 1977, with the aim of establishing an association between genetic, immunologic and microbial factors in MS aetiology and pathogenesis, Ellison *et al.* [106] began a study covering all these factors, in which they found a weak association between high anti-VCA antibody titres and the HLA-DW2 molecule expression in patients with the disease, something absent in the control population. In 1986, Compston *et al.* [107] carried out another study in which they found a significant relationship between a high rate of anti-EBV antibodies and HLA-DR2 in patients. More recently, Nielsen *et al.* [108] did research on the relationship between HLADRB1*1501 alleles, IM and MS, and found that in allele-carrier patients that do not have IM, the risk of developing MS was 2.4 times higher versus healthy controls, and that this risk increased seven-fold in persons with a history of IM.

Sündstrom *et al.* [109] proved that the risk of developing MS was higher in persons with anti-EBNA1 and HLA DRB1*1501 positivity. Later, in another study, Sündstrom *et al.* [110] considered the epitopic reactivity of antibodies against specific EBNA1 fragments and their association with HLA DRB1*1501 molecule, observing that MS patients showed a higher epitopic reactivity against several EBNA1 domains in comparison to controls. They determined that the association of HLA DRB1*1501 expression with the presence of anti-EBNA1 antibodies increases the risk of developing MS 24 fold. HLA DRB1*1501 positivity may be related to an increase in the ability of the immune system to recognize EBNA1 in MS patients.

Conclusions

Therefore, and considering all the publications analyzed, a statistically significant association exists between EBV infection and MS, demonstrated by a higher serum prevalence of anti-VCA IgG antibodies, anti-EBNA complex IgG, heterophile antibodies and, particularly, anti-EBNA1 IgG in patients with the disease, but the study of the presence of virus DNA in serum, cerebrospinal fluid or brain tissue shows no association. Considering that this association was established from the detection of markers that mainly indicate a past infection, not from those that indicate acute infection or exacerbation, we think that infection by this virus may be due to an environmental factor, together with other environmental and endogenous factors, that influences at the earliest stages, thus altering the normal immune function, generating inflammation and demyelination and favouring the start of the disease pathogenesis.

This important relationship found between the disease and the presence of EBV antibodies may suggest their potential value as markers for early diagnosis and follow up of multiple sclerosis.

However, we are of the opinion that there is need for new prospective and comparative studies involving a sufficient number of patients, using a combination of several micro-biological techniques for a same subject and sample, and, most importantly, deter-mining the different viral infection markers and assessing the clinical situation of the patient, especially years before the appearance of the first MS symptoms.

References

[1] Leibowitz, U; Antonovsky, A; Medalie, JM; Smith, HA; Halpern, L; Alter, M. Epidemiological study of multiple sclerosis in Israel. II. Multiple sclerosis and level of sanitation. *J. Neurol. Neurosurg. Psychiatry.*, 1966, 29, 60-8.

[2] Ascherio, A. Epstein-Barr virus in the development of multiple sclerosis. *Expert Rev. Neurother.*, 2008, 8, 331-3.

[3] Kurtzke, JF. Epidemiologic evidence for multiple sclerosis as an infection. *Clin. Microbiol. Rev.*, 1993, 6, 382-427.

[4] Ascherio, A; Munger, KL. Environmental risk factors for multiple sclerosis. Part I: the role of infection. *Ann. Neurol.*, 2007, 61, 288-99.

[5] Giovannoni, G; Ebers, G. Multiple sclerosis: the environment and causation. *Curr. Opin. Neurol.*, 2007, 20, 361-8.

[6] Warner, HB; Carp, RI. Multiple sclerosis and Epstein–Barr virus. *Lancet*, 1981, 318, 1290.

[7] Alonso, A; Egües Olazabal, N; Ayo Martin, O. Infection by Epstein-Barr virus and multiple sclerosis. *Neurologia*, 2006, 21, 249-55.

[8] Haahr, S; Höllsberg, P. Multiple sclerosis is linked to Epstein-Barr virus infection. *Rev. Med. Viro.*, 2006, 16, 297-310.

[9] Riise, T; Gronning, M; Klauber, MR; Barrett-Connor, E; Nyland, H; Albrektsen, G. Clustering of residence of multiple sclerosis patients at age 13 to 20 years in Hordaland, Norway. *Am. J. Epidemiol.*, 1991, 133, 932-9.

[10] Grant, WB. Hypothesis-ultraviolet-B irradiance and vitamin D reduce the risk of viral infections and thus their sequelae, including autoimmune diseases and some cancers. *Photochem. Photobiol.*, 2008, 84, 356-65.

[11] Douglas, AS; Brown, T; Reid, D. Infectious mononucleosis and Hodgkin's disease-a similar seasonality. *Leuk. Lymphoma*, 1996, 23, 323-31.

[12] Goldacre, MJ; Wotton, CJ; Seagroatt, V; Yeates, D. Multiple sclerosis after infectious mononucleosis: record linkage study. *J. Epidemiol. Community Health*, 2004, 58, 1032-5.

[13] Haahr, S; Plesner, AM; Vestergaard, BF; Höllsberg, P. A role of late Epstein–Barr virus infection in multiple sclerosis. *Acta Neurol. Scand.*, 2004, 109, 270-5.

[14] Haahr, S; Koch-Henriksen, N; Moller-Larsen, A; Eriksen, LS; Andersen, HM. Increased risk of multiple sclerosis after late Epstein-Barr virus infection: a historical prospective study. *Mult. Scler.*, 1995, 1, 73-7.

[15] Hernan, MA; Zhang, SM; Lipworth, L; Olek, MJ; Ascherio, A. Multiple sclerosis and age at infection with common viruses. *Epidemiology*, 2001, 12, 301-6.

[16] Lindberg, C; Andersen, O; Vahlne, A; Dalton, M; Runmarker, B. Epidemiological investigation of the association between infectious mononucleosis and multiple sclerosis. *Neuroepidemiology*, 1991, 10, 62-5.

[17] Nielsen, TR; Rostgaard, K; Nielsen, NM; Koch-Henriksen, N; Haahr, S; Sorensen, PS; Hjalgrim, H. Multiple sclerosis after infectious mononucleosis. *Arch. Neurol.*, 2007, 64, 72-5.

[18] Operskalski, EA; Visscher, BR; Malmgren, RM; Detels, R. A case-control study of multiple sclerosis. *Neurology*, 1989, 39, 825-9.

[19] Thacker, EL; Mirzaei, F; Ascherio, A. Infectious mononucleosis and risk for multiple sclerosis: A meta-analysis. *Ann. Neurol.*, 2006, 59, 499-503.

[20] Bray, PF; Luka, J; Culp, KW; Schlight JP. Antibodies against Epstein-Barr nuclear antigen (EBNA) in multiple sclerosis CSF, and two pentapeptide sequence identities between EBNA and myelin basic protein. *Neurology*, 1992, 42, 1798-1804.

[21] Holmoy, T; Kvale, EO; Vartdal, F. Cerebrospinal fluid CD4+ T cells from a multiple sclerosis patient cross-recognize Epstein–Barr virus and myelin basic protein. *J. Neurovirology*, 2004, 10, 278-83.

[22] Lang, HL, Jacobsen, H; Ikemizu, S; Andersson, C; Harlos, K; Madsen, L; Hjorth, P; Sondergaard, L; Svejgaard, A; Wucherpfennig, K; Stuart, DI; Bell, JI; Jones, EY, Fugger, L. A functional and structural basis for TCR cross-reactivity in multiple sclerosis. *Nat. Immunol.*, 2002, 3, 940-3.

[23] Lünemann, JD; Jelcić, I; Roberts, S; Lutterotti, A; Tackenberg, B; Martin, R; Münz, C. EBNA1-specific T cells from patients with multiple sclerosis cross react with myelin antigens and co-produce IFN-gamma and IL-2. *J. Exp. Med.*, 2008, 205, 1763-73.

[24] Vaughan, JH; Riise, T; Rhodes, GH; Nguyen, MD; Barrett-Connor, E; Nyland, H. An Epstein Barr virus-related cross reactive autoimmune response in multiple sclerosis in Norway. *J. Neuroimmunol.*, 1996, 69, 95-102.

[25] Wucherpfennig, KW; Strominger, JL. Molecular mimicry in T cell-mediated autoimmunity: viral peptides activate human T cell clones specific for myelin basic protein. *Cell*, 1995, 80, 695-705.

[26] Lünemann, JD; Edwards, N; Muraro, PA; Hayashi, S; Cohen, JI; Münz, C; Martin, R. Increased frequency and broadened specificity of latent EBV nuclear antigen-1-specific T cells in multiple sclerosis. *Brain*, 2006, 129, 1493-506.

[27] Lünemann, JD; Kamradt, T; Martin, R; Münz, C. Epstein-Barr virus: Environmental trigger of Multiple Sclerosis? *J. Virol.*, 2007, 81, 6777-84.

[28] Höllsberg, P; Hansen, HJ; Haahr, S. Altered CD8+ T cell responses to selected Epstein-Barr virus immunodominant epitopes in patients with multiple sclerosis. *Clin. Exp. Immunol.*, 2003, 132, 137-43.

[29] Gran, B; Hemmer, B; Vergelli, M; McFarland, HF; Martin, R. Molecular mimicry and multiple sclerosis: degenerate T-cell recognition and the induction of autoimmunity. *Ann. Neurol.*, 1999, 45, 559-67.

[30] Pender, MP. Infection of autoreactive B lymphocytes with EBV, causing chronic autoimmune diseases. *Trends Immunol.*, 2003, 24, 584-8.

[31] Kilger, E; Kieser, A; Baumann, M; Hammerschmidt, W. Epstein-Barr virus-mediated B-cell proliferation is dependent upon latent membrane protein 1, which simulates an activated CD40 receptor. *EMBO J.*, 1998, 17, 1700-9.

[32] Mosialos, G; Birkenbach, M; Yalamanchili, R; VanArsdale, T; Ware, C; Kieff, E. The Epstein-Barr virus transforming protein LMP1 engages signalling proteins for the tumor necrosis factor receptor family. *Cell*, 1995, 80, 389-99.

[33] Thorley-Lawson, DA. Epstein-Barr virus: exploiting the immune system. *Nat. Rev. Immunol.*, 2001, 1, 75-82.

[34] Middeldorp, JM, Brink, AA, van den Brule, AJ; Meijer, CJ. Pathogenic roles for Epstein-Barr virus (EBV) gene products in EBV-associated proliferative disorders. *Crit. Rev. Oncol. Hematol.*, 2003, 45, 1-36.

[35] Desbien, AL; Kappler, JW; Marrack, P. The Epstein-Barr virus Bcl-2 homolog, BHRF1, blocks apoptosis by binding to a limited amount of Bim. *Proc, Natl, Acad, Sci, USA*, 2009, 106, 5663-8.

[36] Henderson, S; Huen, D; Rowe, M; Dawson, C; Johnson, G; Rickinson, A. Epstein-Barr virus-coded BHRF1 protein, a viral homologue of Bcl-2, protects human B cells from programmed cell death. *Proc. Natl. Acad. Sci. USA*, 1993, 90, 8479-83.

[37] Uchida, J; Yasui, T; Takaoka-Shichijo, Y; Muraoka, M; Kulwichit, W; Raab-Traub, N; Kikutani, H. Mimicry of CD40 signals by Epstein-Barr virus LMP1 in B lymphocyte responses. *Science*, 1999, 286, 300-3.

[38] Levitskaya, J; Coram, M; Levitsky, V; Imreh, S; Steigerwald-Mullen, PM; Klein, G; Kurilla, MG; Masucci, MG. Inhibition of antigen processing by the internal repeat region of the Epstein-Barr virus antigen-1. *Nature*, 1995, 375, 685-8.

[39] Qin, Y; Duquette, P; Zhang, Y; Talbot, P; Poole, R; Antel, J. Clonal expansion and somatic hypermutation of V(H) genes of B cells from cerebrospinal fluid in multiple sclerosis. *J. Clin. Invest.*, 1998, 102, 1045-50.

[40] Colombo, M; Dono, M; Gazzola, P; Chiorazzi, N; Mancardi, G, Ferrarini, M. Maintenance of B lymphocyte-related clones in the cerebrospinal fluid of multiple sclerosis patients. *Eur. J. Immunol.*, 2003, 33, 3433-8.

[41] Walsh, MJ, Tourtellotte, WW. Temporal invariance and clonal uniformity of brain and cerebrospinal IgG, IgA, and IgM in multiple sclerosis. *J. Exp. Med.*, 1986, 163, 41-53.

[42] Cepok, S; Zhou, D; Srivastava, R; Nessler, S, Stei, S; Büssow, K; Sommer, N; Hemmer, B. Identification of Epstein-Barr virus proteins as putative targets of the immune response in multiple sclerosis. *J. Clin. Invest.*, 2005, 115, 1352-60.

[43] Reiber, H; Peter, JB. Cerebrospinal fluid analysis: disease-related data patterns and evaluation programs. *J. Neurol. Sci.*, 2001, 184, 101-22.

[44] Sindic, CJ; Monteyne, P; Laterre, EC. The intrathecal synthesis of virus-specific oligoclonal IgG in multiple sclerosis. *J. Neuroimmunol.*, 1994, 54, 75-80.

[45] Serafini, B; Rosicarelli, B; Franciotta, D; Magliozzi, R; Reynolds, R; Cinque, P; Andreoni, L; Trivedi, P; Salvetti, M; Faggioni, A; Aloisi, F. Dysregulated Epstein-Barr virus infection in the multiple sclerosis brain. *J. Exp. Med.*, 2007, 204, 2899-912.

[46] Wucherpfennig, KW; Catz, I; Hausmann, S; Strominger, JL; Steinman, L; Warren, KG. Recognition of the immunodominantmyelin basic protein peptide by autoantibodies and HLA DR2-restricted T cell clones from multiple sclerosis patients. Identity of key contact residues in the B-cell and T-cell epitopes. *J. Clin. Invest.*, 1997, 100, 1114-22.

[47] Torkildsen, O; Stansberg, C; Angelskår, SM; Kooi, EJ; Geurts, JJ; van der Valk, P; Myhr, KM; Steen, VM; Bø, L. Upregulation of immunoglobulin-related genes in cortical sections from multiple sclerosis patients. *Brain Pathol.*, 2010, 20, 720-9.

[48] Willis, SN; Stadelmann, C; Rodig, SJ; Caron, T; Gattenloehner, S; Mallozzi, SS; Roughan, JE; Almendinger, SE; Blewett, MM; Brück, W; Hafler, DA; O'Connor, KC. Epstein-Barr virus infection is not a characteristic feature of multiple sclerosis brain. *Brain*, 2009, 132, 3318-28.

[49] Haahr, S; Sommerlund, M; Moller-Larsen, A; Mogensen, S; Andersen, HM. Is multiple sclerosis caused by a dual infection with retrovirus and Epstein-Barr virus? *Neuroepidemiology*, 1992, 11, 299-303.

[50] Sutkowski, N; Palkama, T; Ciurli, C; Sekaly, RP; Thorley-Lawson, DA; Huber, BT; An Epstein-Barr virus-asociated superantigen. *J. Exp. Med.*, 1996, 184, 971-80.

[51] Angius, MA; Kirvan, CA; Schafer, AL; Gudipati, E; Zhu, S. High prevalence of anti-alpha-crystallin antibodies in multiple sclerosis: correlation with severity and activity of disease. *Acta Neurol. Scand.*, 1999, 100, 139-47.

[52] Ousman, SS; Tomooka, BH; van Noort, JM; Wawrousek, EF; O'Connor, KC; Hafler, DA; Sobel, RA; Robinson, WH; Steinman, L. Protective and therapeutic role for alpha B-crystallin in autoimmune demyelination. *Nature*, 2007, 448, 474-9.

[53] van Noort, JM; van Sechel, AC; Bajramovic, JJ; Bajramovic, JJ. The small heat-shock protein alpha B-crystallin as candidate autoantigen in multiple sclerosis. *Nature*, 1995, 375, 798-801.

[54] van Sechel, AC; Bajramovic, JJ; van Noort, JM. EBV-induced expression and HLA-DR restricted presentation by human B cells of alpha B-crystallin, a candidate autoantigen in multiple sclerosis. *J. Immunol.*, 1999, 162, 129-35.

[55] Fleming, J; Fabry, Z. The hygiene hypothesis and multiple sclerosis. *Ann. Neurol.*, 2007, 61, 85-8.

[56] Bach, JF. The effect of infections on susceptibility to autoimmune and allergic diseases. *N. Eng. J. Med.*, 2002, 347, 911-20.

[57] Krone, B; Oeffner, F; Grange, JM. Is the risk of multiple sclerosis related to the 'biography' of the immune system? *J. Neurol.*, 2009, 256, 1052-60.

[58] Sundstedt, A; O'Neill, EJ; Nicolson, KS; Wraith, DC. Role for IL-10 in suppression mediated by peptide induced regulatory T cells in vivo. *J. Immunol.*, 2003, 170, 1240-8.

[59] Viglietta, V; Baecher-Allan, C; Weiner, HL; Hafler, DA. Loss of functional suppression by CD4+ CD25+ regulatory T cells in patients with multiple sclerosis. *J. Exp. Med.*, 2004, 199, 971-9.

[60] Ablashi, DV, Lapps, W; Kaplan, M; Whitman, JE; Richert, JR; Pearson, GR. Human herpesvirus-6 (HHV-6). Infection in multiple sclerosis: a preliminary report. *Mult. Scler.*, 1998, 4, 490-6.

[61] Alotaibi, S; Kennnedy, J; Tellier, R; Stephens, D; Banwell, B. Epstein-barr virus in pediatric multiple sclerosis. *JAMA*, 2004, 291, 1875-9.

[62] Alvarez, R; Cour, I; Kankan, A; Benedicto, M; Martin-Estefania, C; Arroyo, R; Varela de Seijas, E; Picazo, JJ. Detection of viral genomes of the *Herpesviridae* family in multiple sclerosis patients by means of the polymerase chain reaction (PCR). *Enferm. Infecc. Microbiol. Clin.*, 2000, 18, 223-8.

[63] Alvarez-Lafuente, R; Garcia-Montojo, M, De Las Heras, V; Dominguez-Mozo, MI; Bartolome, M; Benito-Martin, MS; Arroyo, R. Herpesviruses and human endogenous retroviral sequences in the cerebrospinal fluid of multiple sclerosis patients. *Mult. Scler.*, 2008, 14, 595-601.

[64] Ascherio, A; Munger, KL; Lennette, ET; Spiegelman, D; Hernán, MA; Olek, MJ; Hankinson, SE; Hunter, DJ. Epstein-barr virus antibodies and risk of multiple sclerosis. *JAMA*, 2001, 286, 3083-8.

[65] Banwell, B; Krupp, L; Kennedy, J; Tellier, R; Tenembaum, S; Ness, J; Belman, A; Boiko, A; Bykova, O; Waubant, E; Mah, JK; Stoian, C; Kremenchutzky, M; Bardini, MR; Ruggieri, M; Rensel, M; Hahn, J; Weinstock-Guttman, B; Yeh, EA; Farrell, K; Freedman, M; Iivanainen, M; Sevon, M; Bhan, V; Dilenge, ME; Stephens, D; Bar-Or, A. Clinical features and virologies in children with multiple sclerosis: a multinational observational study. *Lancet Neurol.*, 2007, 6, 773-81.

[66] Bray, PF; Bloomer, LC; Salmon, VC; Bagley, MH; Larsen, PD. Epstein-barr virus infection and antibody synthesis in patients with multiple sclerosis. *Arch. Neurol.*, 1983, 40, 406-8.

[67] Buljevac, D; van Doornum, GJ; Flach, HZ; Groen, J; Osterhaus, AD; Hop, W; van Doorn, PA; van der Meché, FG; Hintzen, RQ. Epstein-Barr virus and disease activity in multiple sclerosis. *J. Neurol. Neurosurg. Psychiatry.*, 2005, 76, 1377-81.

[68] Denne, C; Kleines, M; Dieckhofer, A; Ritter, K; Scheithauer, S; Merz, U; Häusler, M. Intrathecal synthesis of anti-viral antibodies in pediatric patients. *Eur. J. Paediatr. Neurol.*, 2007, 11, 29-34.

[69] Ferrante, P; Mancuso, R; Pagani, E; Guerini, FR; Calvo, MG; Saresella, M; Speciale, L; Caputo, D. Molecular evidences for a role of HSV-1 in multiple sclerosis clinical acute attack. *J. Neurovirol.*, 2000, 6, S109-14.

[70] Gutierrez, J; Vergara, MJ; Guerrero, M; Fernandez, O; Piedrola, G; Morales, P; Maroto, MC. Multiple sclerosis and human herpesvirus 6. *Infection*, 2002, 30, 145-9.

[71] Hay, KA, Tenser, RB. Leukotropic herpesviruses in multiple sclerosis. *Mult. Scler.*, 2000, 6, 66-8.

[72] Höllsberg, P; Kusk, M; Bech, E; Hansen, HJ; Jakobsen, J; Haahr, S. Presence of Epstein-Barr virus and human herpesvirus 6B in multiple sclerosis patients: associations with clinical activity. *Acta Neurol. Scand.*, 2005, 112, 395-402.

[73] Larsen, PD; Bloomer, LC; Bray, PF. Epstein-Barr nuclear and viral capsid antigen antibody titers in multiple sclerosis. *Neurology*, 1985, 35, 435-8.

[74] Mancuso, R; Delbue, S; Borghi, E; Pagani, E, Calvo, MG; Caputo, D; Granieri, E; Ferrante, P. Increased prevalence of varicella zoster virus DNA in cerebrospinal fluid from patients with multiple sclerosis. *J. Med. Virol.*, 2007, 79:192-9.

[75] Martin, C; Enbom, M; Södertröm, M; Fredrikson, S; Dahl, H; Lycke, J; Bergström, T; Linde, A. Absence of seven human herpesviruses including HHV-6, by polymerasa chain reaction in CSF and blood from patients with multiple sclerosis and optic neuritis. *Acta Neurol. Scand.*, 1997, 95, 280-3.

[76] Myhr, KM; Riise, T; Barrett-Connor, E; Myrmel, H; Vedeler, C; Grønning, M, Kalvenes, MB; Nyland H. Altered antibody pattern to Epstein-Barr virus but not to other herpesviruses in multiple sclerosis: a population based case-control study from western Norway. *J. Neurol. Neurosurg. Psychiatry*, 1998, 64, 539-42.

[77] Morre, SA; van Beek, J; De Groot, CJ; Killestein, J; Meijer, CJ; Polman, CH; van der Valk, P; Middeldorp, JM; van Den Brule, AJ. Is Epstein-Barr virus present in the CNS of patients with MS? *Neurology*, 2001, 56, 692.

[78] Munch, M; Riisom, K; Christensen, T; Møller-Larsen, A; Haahr, S. The significance of Epstein-Barr virus seropositivity in multiple sclerosis patients? *Acta Neurol. Scand.*, 1998, 97, 171-4.

[79] Nikoskelainen, E; Nikoskelainen, J; Salmi, AA; Halonen, PE. Virus antibody levels in the cerebrospinal fluid from patients with optic neuritis. *Acta Neurol. Scand.*, 1975, 51, 347-64.

[80] Pohl, D; Krone, B; Rostasy, K; Kahler, E, Brunner, E; Lehnert, M; Wagner, HJ; Gärtner, J; Hanefeld, F. High seroprevalence of Epstein–Barr virus in children with multiple sclerosis. *Neurology*, 2006, 67, 2063-5.

[81] Ponsonby, AL; van der Mei, I; Dwyer, T; Blizzard, L; Taylor, B; Kemp, A; Simmons, R; Kilpatrick, T. Exposure to infant siblings during early life and risk of multiple sclerosis. *JAMA*, 2005, 293, 463-9.

[82] Riverol, M; Sepulcre, J; Fernández-Díez, B; Villoslada, P; Fernández-Alonso, M; Rubio, M; Rodriguez, A; Uccelli, A; Brieva, L. Antibodies against Epstein-Barr virus and herpesvirus type 6 are associated with the early phases of multiple sclerosis. *J. Neuroimmunol.*, 2007, 192, 184-5.

[83] Sanders, VJ; Felisan, S; Waddell, A; Tourtellotte, WW. Detection of herpesviridae in postmortem multiple sclerosis brain tissue and controls by polymerase chain reactión. *J. Neurovirol.*, 1996, 2, 249-58.

[84] Shirodaria, PV; Haire, M; Fleming, E; Merrett, JD; Hawkins, SA; Roberts, SD. Viral antibody titers. Comparison in patients with multiple sclerosis and rheumatoid arthritis. *Arch. Neurol.*, 1987, 44, 1237-41.

[85] Sotelo, J; Ordóñez, G, Pineda, B. Varicella-Zoster virus at relapses of multiple sclerosis. *J. Neurol.*, 2007; 254; 493-500.

[86] Sumaya, CV; Myers, LW; Ellison, GW. Epstein-Barr virus antibodies in multiple sclerosis. *Trans. Am. Neurol. Assoc.*, 1976, 101, 300-2.

[87] Sumaya, CV; Myers, LW; Ellison, GW. Epstein-Brr virus antibodies in multiple sclerosis. *Arch. Neurol.*, 1980, 37, 94-6

[88] Sundström, P; Juto, P; Wadell, G; Hallmans, G; Svenningsson, A; Nyström, L., Dillner, J; Forsgren, L. An altered immune response to Epstein-Barr virus in multiple sclerosis: a prospective study. *Neurology*, 2004, 62, 2277-82.

[89] Wagner, HJ; Munger, KL; Ascherio, A. Plasma viral load of Eptein-Barr virus and risk of multiple sclerosis. *Eur. J. Neurol.*, 2004, 11, 833-4.

[90] Wandinger, KP; Jabs, W; Siekhaus, A; Bubel, S; Trillenberg, P; Wagner, H; Wessel, K; Kirchner, H; Hennig, H. Association between clinical disease activity and Epstein-Barr virus reactivation in MS. *Neurology*, 2000, 55, 178-84.

[91] Zivadinov, R; Nasuelli, D; Tommasi, MA; Serafin, M; Bratina, A; Ukmar, M; Pirko, I; Johnson, AJ, Furlan, C; Pozzi-Mucelli, RS; Monti-Bragadin, L; Grop, A; Zambon, M; Antonello, RM; Cazzato, G; Zorzon M. Positivity of citomegalovirus antibodies predicts a better clinical and radiological outcome in mutiple sclerosis patients. *Neurol. Res.*, 2006, 28, 262-9.

[92] Santiago, O; Gutierrez, J; Sorlozano, A; Luna, JD; Villegas, E; Fernandez, O. Relation between Epstein-Barr virus and multiple sclerosis: analytic study of scientific production. *Eur. J. Clin. Microbiol. Infect. Dis.*, 2010, 29, 857-66.

[93] DeLorenze, GN; Munger, KL; Lennette, ET; Orentreich, N; Vogelman, JH; Ascherio, A. Epstein-Barr virus and multiple sclerosis: evidence of association from a prospective study with long-term follow-up. *Arch. Neurol.*, 2006, 63, 839-44.

[94] Woyciechowska, JL; Dambrozia, J; Leinikki, P; Shekarchi, C; Wallen, W; Sever, J; McFarland, H; McFarlin, D. Viral antibodies in twins with multiple sclerosis. *Neurology*, 1985, 35, 1176-80.

[95] de-The, G; Geser, A; Day, NE; Tukei, PM; Williams, EH; Beri, DP; Smith, PG; Dean, AG; Bronkamm, GW; Feorino, P; Henle W. Epidemiological evidence for causal relationship between Epstein-Barr virus and Burkitt´s lymphoma from Ugandan prospective study. *Nature*, 1978, 274, 756-61.

[96] Zeng, Y. Seroepidemiological studies on nasopharyngeal carcinoma in China. *Adv. Cancer Res.*, 1985, 44, 121-38.

[97] Mueller, N; Evans, A; Harris, NL; Comstock, GW; Jellum, E; Magnus, K; Orentreich, N; Polk, BF; Vogelman, J. Hodgkin´s disease and Epstein-Barr virus: altered antibody pattern before diagnosis. *N. Engl. J. Med.*, 1989, 320, 689-95.

[98] Dölken, G; Bross, KJ; Hecht, T; Brugger, W; Löhr, GW; Hirsch, FW. Increased incidence of IgA antibodies to the Epstein-Barr virus-associated viral capsid antigen

and early antigens in patients with chronic lymphocytic leukemia. *Int. J. Cancer.*, 1986, 38, 55-9.

[99] Origgi, L; Perego, R; Hu, C; Bertetti, E; D'Agostino, P; Asero, R; Riboldi, P. Anti-Epstein-Barr virus antibodies in systemic lupus erythematosus. *Boll. Ist. Sieroter. Milan*, 1988, 67, 116-22.

[100] Zandman-Goddard, G; Berkun, Y; Barzilai, O, Boaz, M; Blank, M; Ram, M; Sherer, Y; Anaya, JM, Shoenfeld, Y. Exposure to Epstein-Barr virus infection is associated with mild systemic lupus erythematosus disease. *Ann. N. Y. Acad. Sci.*, 2009, 1173, 658-63.

[101] Yao, QY; Rickinson, AB; Gaston, JS; Epstein, MA. In vitro analysis of the Epstein-Barr virus: host balance in long-term renal allograft recipients. *Int. J. Cancer*, 1985, 35, 43-9.

[102] Yao, QY; Tierney, RJ, Croom-Carter, D; Dukers, D; Cooper, GM; Ellis, CJ; Rowe, M; Rickinson, AB. Frequency of multiple Epstein-Barr virus infections in T cell-immunocompromised individuals. *J. Virol.*, 1996, 70, 4884-94.

[103] Gutierrez, J; Sorlozano, A; Soto, MJ; Maroto, C. Microbiological diagnosis of infection by the Epstein-Barr virus: pathogenic basis. In: New developments in Epstein-Barr virus research. Columbus F (ed.). New York, USA. Nova Biomedical Books; 2006.

[104] Levin, LI; Munger, KL; Rubertone, MV; Peck, CA; Lennette, ET; Spiegelman, D; Ascherio, A. Multiple sclerosis and Epstein–Barr virus. *JAMA*, 2003, 289, 1533-6.

[105] Levin, LI; Munger, KL; Rubertone, MV; Peck, CA; Lennette, ET; Spiegelman, D; Ascherio, A. Temporal relationship between elevation of Eptein-Barr virus antibody titers and initial onset of neurological symptoms in multiple sclerosis. *JAMA*, 2005, 293, 2496-500

[106] Ellison, GW; Myers, LW; Sumaya, CV; Terasaki, PI; Opelz, G; Holevoet, MI. Epstein-Barr virus antibodies and histocompatibility type in multiple sclerosis. *Trans. Am. Neurol. Assoc.*, 1977, 102, 59-60.

[107] Compston, DA; Vakarelis, BN; Paul, E; McDonald, WI; Batchelor, JR; Mims, CA. Viral infection in patients with multiple sclerosis and HLA-DR matched controls. *Brain*, 1986, 109, 325-44.

[108] Nielsen, TR; Rostgaard, K; Askling, J; Steffensen, R; Oturai, A; Jersild, C; Koch-Henriksen, N; Sørensen, PS; Hjalgrim, H. Effects of infectious mononucleosis and HLA-DRB1*15 in multiple sclerosis. *Mult. Scler.*, 2009, 15, 431-6.

[109] Sundström, P; Nyström, L; Jidell, E; Hallmans, G. EBNA-1 reactivity and HLA DRB1*1501 as statistically independent risk factors for multiple sclerosis: a case–control study. *Mult. Scler.*, 2008, 14, 1120-2.

[110] Sundström, P; Nyström, L; Ruuth, K; Lundgren, E. Antibodies to specific EBNA-1 domains and HLA DRB1*1501 interact as risk factors for multiple sclerosis. *J. Neuroimmunol.*, 2009, 215, 102-7.

In: Multiple Sclerosis
Editor: E. Scholz and C. Müller, pp. 113-130
ISBN 978-1-61324-848-5

Chapter VI

MR Diffusion Tensor Imaging in Multiple Sclerosis: A Regional and Statistical Analysis of Microstructural Alterations

Dominique Sappey-Marinier,[1,2,*] ***Salem Hannoun,***[1]
Françoise Durand-Dubief,[1,3]
François Cotton,[1] ***Christian Confavreux***[3]
[1]CREATIS, UMR5220 CNRS & U1044 INSERM, Université de Lyon, Villeurbanne, France
[2]MRI Department, CERMEP-Imagerie du Vivant, Groupement Hospitalier Est, Bron, France
[3]Service de Neurologie A, Hôpital Neurologique, Groupement Hospitalier Est, Bron, France

Abstract

Magnetic Resonance Imaging (MRI) became the first radiological examination that is essential to the diagnosis of Multiple Sclerosis (MS), and most informative for the understanding of the illness and the patient care. If conventional MRI shows the lesion load reflecting mainly the inflammatory aspect of the disease, the lack of clinico-radiological correlation has led to the research of new markers for monitoring and predicting the progression of the disease to better adapt the medical treatment to each patient. Therefore, quantitative MR methods have been developed to better access these

* Corresponding author: Dominique Sappey-Marinier, PhD. Address: Département IRM, CERMEP-Imagerie du Vivant, Groupement Hospitalier Est - 59, Boulevard Pinel - 69677 Bron, France. Tel: +33 4 72 68 86 07 ; Fax: + 33 4 72 68 86 10; E-mail: Dominique.Sappey-Marinier@univ-lyon1.fr.
Grant Support: Clinical Research Hospital Program (PHRC 2004) from French Government Health Minister and Rhône-Alpes Region.

alterations that were undetectable by conventional MRI such as diffusion tensor imaging (DTI). DTI is a very promising technique for fiber tracking the cerebral white matter (WM) as well as to provide accurate quantification of biophysic markers reflecting microstructure alterations of axonal/neuronal integrity and connectivity. This information can be obtained through the measurement of several parameters such as the fractional anisotropy (FA), the mean diffusivity (MD) and the axial and radial diffusivities (λa and λr) by selecting regions of interest (ROI) in lesions, normal appearing WM or structures such as the corpus callosum. More recently, the ability to analyze DTI data in a voxelwise approach using statistic techniques such "Tract-Based Spatial Statistics" (TBSS) allowed us to localize alterations in an observer-independent manner in the whole WM of patients with different clinical forms.

Therefore, to investigate the role of DTI for better characterizing the pathological processes in different clinical forms of MS, we performed a study on 69 patients with Relapsing Remitting (RR), primary (PP) and secondary progressive (SP) and 29 control subjects. The quantification of DTI metrics demonstrated significant increases of MD, λa, and λr, and a decrease of FA in MS patients of any clinical form compared to control subjects. Moreover, these alterations were significantly greater in progressive forms such SP and PP compared to RR. Compared to FA and λa, the radial diffusivity showed the best sensitivity to detect alterations. This result may suggest a better specificity of this marker to the demyelinating and inflammatory processes. As shown by both ROI and TBSS approaches, the corpus callosum appeared the most and earliest damaged structure in RR patients, probably due to inflammatory attacks as confirmed by the good correlation obtained between DTI values and the lesion load. Therefore, DTI metrics constitute an early and sensitive marker to follow-up the white matter alterations and better understand the disease progression.

Keywords: Multiple Sclerosis, Diffusion Tensor Imaging, White Matter, inflammation, lesion load, anisotropy, diffusivity

Introduction

Magnetic resonance imaging (MRI) completely changed brain diseases perception and allows today the improvement of patient care by specifying diagnosis, lesion localization and extension, and therapeutic follow-up. Besides, functional and metabolic MR modalities, along with quantitative and statistical processing methods, bring new fundamental information for a better understanding of pathological processes. These prospective approaches are essential in the survey of multiple sclerosis (MS). While MS constitutes the first cause of non-traumatic handicap in young adults, therapeutic management is only guided by the patient clinical evolution that remains a challenge to predict. The disease may appear either as a clinically isolated syndrome (CIS), a relapsing-remittent (RR) phase of inflammation which will be sooner or later followed by a secondary progressive (SP) period or directly as a primary progressive (PP) evolution [1]. Since the discovery of lesions by Charcot et al. [2], MS has been considered a white matter (WM) disease characterized by inflammatory acute phases of demyelination followed either by variable remyelination or further axonal degeneration in chronic lesions.

Conventional MRI

The ability of MRI to detect subclinical lesions has led to its widespread acceptance as an essential tool in the diagnostic work-up [3] as well as in obtaining prognostic information in the course of the disease [4]. In addition, screening of new MS therapies has been largely improved by the use of MRI which provides sensitive and reproducible measures of the disease burden through the assessment of hyper-intensities on T2-weighted images and on gadolinium (Gd) enhanced T1-weighted images. While Gd-enhanced MRI is very sensitive for the detection of active and deep WM lesions, T2-weighted MRI shows large periventricular regions of hyperintensities, reflecting increased water content, focal demyelination and axonal loss to variable extents [5-6] that are poorly correlated with the clinical status of the patient. In contrast, T1-hypointense lesions, also known as "back holes", can better predict disability progression, suggesting axonal damage [7].

However, MS pathological hallmark is not limited to WM lesions. First, the micro-architecture of normal appearing WM (NAWM) is also altered by diffuse damage including inflammation and microglial reactions, and neurodegeneration as demonstrated by histological studies [8-9]. Second, there is increasing evidence for grey matter (GM) pathology in MS. Since the pioneers pathological studies dating back to the 19th century [10] and more recently, the use of sensitive immuno-histochemical techniques [11], cortical and subcortical GM lesions have been identified and classified as type I (cortical-juxtacortical), type II (vascular cortical), and type III (subpial) lesions [12]. If these cortical lesions may constitute the basis of neurologic impairments in MS patients, they remained undetectable by conventional clinical MRI due to both limited tissue contrast and spatial resolution. Further, the modest correlation observed between the lesion load, as measured by conventional MRI, and the patient clinical status, has led to the concept of "clinico-radiological paradox", and has contributed to the emergence of the neurodegenerative hypothesis implying diffuse and microscopic axonal damages [13]. Therefore, quantitative and more advanced MR methods have been developed to better characterize diffuse tissue damage. These non-conventional MR techniques include diffusion tensor imaging (DTI) that can explore the biophysical properties of water molecules motion in the brain and provide information on tissue microarchitecture.

Diffusion Tensor Imaging

Based on the measurement of water molecules Brownian motion, the story of diffusion MRI has started shortly after Bloch and Purcell discovery of the Nuclear Magnetic Resonance (NMR) phenomenon. In 1950, Hahn published the pioneer sequence of spin-echo that did not only constitute the basic sequence of MRI but also demonstrated that the NMR signal is reduced by the random thermal motion of the spins in the presence of magnetic field homogeneity. This fundamental notion for the understanding of diffusion MRI has led in 1965 to the initial gradient spin-echo sequence of Stejskal and Tanner [14] (Figure 1).

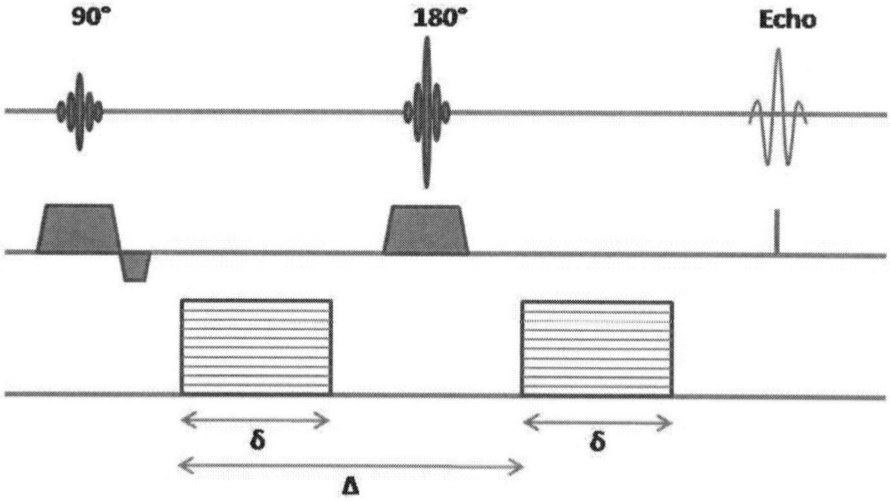

Figure 1. Stejskal and Tanner spin-echo sequence used to measure water molecules diffusion in a direction given by the gradient. This sequence is composed of two gradient pulses, applied for a duration time δ and separated by a time Δ, placed before and after the 180° refocusing pulse. The first gradient pulse causes a phase shift of the spins while the combination of the 180° pulse and the second gradient induces an inverse second phase shift that cancels the first phase shift only for the static spins. In contrast, spins under Brownian motion during the time period Δ experience different phase shifts resulting in a T2 signal attenuation in q-space where the value of q is given by $q= \gamma\delta G/2\pi$ with γ the nuclear gyromagnetic ratio for water protons and G the applied diffusion gradient vector.

These principle developments have led in 1985 to the initial experiments of diffusion-weighted imaging (DWI) [15] that were applied in human brain by Le Bihan et al. [16]. These images allowed measuring the average diffusion coefficient (ADC) as given by the simplified equation:

$$ADC = -\frac{1}{b} ln\left(\frac{S}{S_0}\right)$$

based on the assumption that the probability density function of diffusion displacement is Gaussian and where b is the diffusion-weighted value. Following Moseley et al. [17] experiment using strong diffusion gradients to demonstrate the presence of cytotoxic edema induced immediately after occlusion in cat brain in 1990, DWI became the reference method for the clinical evaluation of acute stroke [18] and also one of the most sensitive brain MRI method. If Douek et al. [19] suggested that diffusion MRI can measure the ADC in two directions to determine orientations of fibers bundles in white matter, the dependency of these measurements on the direction of the acquisition gradient led to the search of a new rotationally invariant method. In 1992, Basser et al. [20] proposed the use of a tensor to model the diffusion properties in biological tissue.

Based on the previous assumption that the diffusion probability has a normal distribution (Gaussian) in the 3 directions of space, the diffusion coefficient D can be replaced by a diffusion tensor (DT):

$$D = \begin{pmatrix} D_{xx} & D_{xy} & D_{xz} \\ D_{yx} & D_{yy} & D_{yz} \\ D_{zx} & D_{zy} & D_{zz} \end{pmatrix} = \begin{pmatrix} \lambda_1 & 0 & 0 \\ 0 & \lambda_2 & 0 \\ 0 & 0 & \lambda_3 \end{pmatrix} \begin{pmatrix} \varepsilon_1 \\ \varepsilon_2 \\ \varepsilon_3 \end{pmatrix}$$

Since D is symmetric, only six unknown coefficients would be estimated, requiring only 6 acquisitions instead of nine, and one acquisition without diffusion gradient. Typically, a b-value of 1000 s/mm^2 is used with 6 to 60 gradient directions in clinical brain acquisitions. First of all, the DT can be decomposed into its three eigenvalues λ1, λ2, λ3 where λ1>λ2>λ3 and the corresponding eigenvectors e1, e2, e3, where the largest eigenvalue λ1 gives the principal direction (e1) being orthogonal to the plane formed by e2 and e3. Based on the measured eigenvalues, several rotationally invariant metrics can be extracted such as the trace (Tr = λ1+λ2+λ3), the mean diffusivity (MD = Tr/3), the fractional anisotropy (FA) and other measures [21]. Furthermore, the analysis of the axial (λa=λ1) and radial (λr=(λ2+λ3)/2) diffusivity values may bring some insight into the different processes occurring in WM damage. The FA measurement [22] has been extensively used for lesion characterization in many clinical applications. The use of a red-green-blue (RGB) color map indicating the direction of the principal fibers bundles has led to the 3-dimensionnal reconstruction methods of fiber-tracking [23] which constitutes to-day a large domain of research on brain connectivity. However, the DT model is limited because of the Gaussian assumption of diffusion and the limited number of freedom degrees. Hence, new and higher order models such as high angular resolution diffusion imaging (HARDI) [24] and diffusion spectrum imaging (DSI) [25] were developed and were able to better describe "crossing fibers" architecture. Nevertheless, these methods remained unapplied clinical routines due to their long acquisition time and intensive computational requirements.

DTI in Multiple Sclerosis

Initially DWI and more recently DTI have proved to be a very sensitive method to detect microscopic structural changes occurring in lesions and NAWM of MS patients [26-27]. Studies have demonstrated abnormal MD and FA values in lesions [28-29] that may differ between Gd-enhancing versus non-enhancing lesions [30-31]. However, most of these studies showed higher MD and lower FA values in lesions than in NAWM [32] with the extreme values being found in the non-enhanced T1-hypointense lesions. Further, these diffusivity and anisotropy alterations were also observed in NAWM of MS patients when compared to normal controls demonstrating the sensitivity of DTI to detect changes in cell integrity. Indeed, a gradient of FA was observed between the lesion and the surrounding NAWM [33-34]. These findings demonstrate that lesions and NAWM tissue are subject to microstructural alterations as shown by T2-hyperintensities and T1-hypointensities such as disruption of membrane barriers and axonal damage, respectively. These structural changes are probably related to demyelination/remyelination mechanisms, cell proliferation induced by inflammation and neurodegenerative processes [26]. Considering the different clinical forms of MS, DTI findings showed greater changes of MD and FA values in patients with progressive forms such PP and SP suggesting a relation between these markers and the severity of the disease. Furthermore, the main advantage of DTI is to provide quantification of diffusivity values in the three directions of water displacement. As proposed by Lowe et al. [35] the increased radial diffusivity change may be a sensitive marker of myelin porosity and demyelination while the axial diffusivity may better reflect axonal tract damage.

While previous studies were mostly based on region of interest (ROI) approach, the emergence of more advanced imaging processing tools such as voxel-based-morphometry (VBM) for T1-weighted MRI data has provided the ability to perform statistical analysis in an observer-independent manner and free of cerebral region hypothesis. To analyze DTI data in a voxelwise approach, tract-based spatial statistics (TBSS) was recently developed [36]. Based on the determination of the major WM tracts from the FA map, TBSS minimizes registration errors and provides a statistical analysis of the whole brain WM. Recently applied in MS patients, this method can provide a complete brain analysis of all DTI metrics in an objective and quantitative way [37].

Therefore, we proposed in this study to analyze regionaly the microstructural changes detected by DTI using both quantitative ROI and statistic voxelwise approaches. The alterations found in DTI metrics such FA, axial and radial diffusivities will be correlated with the lesion load and the clinical status to better understand the link between these markers and the underlying pathological processes.

Materials and Methods

Subjects

Sixty nine patients (27 RR, 25 SP and 17 PP) (mean age = 39.1 ± 6.8 years) with clinically definite MS according to the McDonald's criteria [3] were included in this study (Table 1). All patients underwent a full neurological examination, and their expended disability status scale (EDSS) was lower than 6. Twenty-five volunteers (mean age = 35.3 ± 10.0 years) with no history of neurological disorders served as control subjects. Local ethical committee approval and written informed consent from all patients and control subjects were obtained prior to study initiation.

Table 1. Demographics and group characteristics

	Controls	RR	SP	PP
Number of subjects	29	27	25	17
Mean age (SD) [years]	36.55 (9.57)	35.13 (7.33)	42.13(4.58)	41.29 (6.74)
Mean disease duration (SD) [years]	-	6.87 (4.16)	14.48 (6.15)	6.93 (2.98)
Mean EDSS (SD)	-	2.50 (1.67)	5.04 (1.18)	4.53 (1.17)
Lesion load	-	0.29 (0.24)	0.61 (0.33)	0.60 (0.41)

RR: relapsing remitting; SP: secondary progressive; PP: primary progressive; EDSS: expanded disability status scale; SD: standard deviation.

MRI Protocol

MRI examinations were performed using a 1.5 Tesla Siemens Sonata system with an 8 elements phased-array head-coil. Conventional MR imaging protocol included a MPR 3D T1-weighted (TR = 1880 ms, TE = 4 ms, TI = 1100 ms) millimetric image of 176 sagittal slices with and without gadolinium injection, a Turbo Spin-Echo (TSE) of proton density (PD) and T2-weighted axial images with 3 mm slice thickness (TR = 3000 ms, TE = 12 ms, 85 ms) and an axial FLAIR image with 3 mm slice thickness (TR = 8000 ms, TE = 105 ms, TI = 2200 ms).

Diffusion tensor spin-echo EPI sequence (TE = 86 ms, TR = 6900 ms) was performed to acquire, 51 axial slices aligned in the anterior commissure - posterior commissure (AC-PC) axis in 24 gradient directions with a 2.5 mm isotropic spatial resolution. Twenty-four volumes with non-collinear diffusion gradients (b = 1000 s/mm2) and 4 volumes without diffusion weighting (b = 0 s/mm2) were obtained using 96 x 96 phase-encodings over a FOV of 240 x 240 mm.

Data Analysis and Post-Processing

Lesion Load Measurement

Lesion load measurement was performed using first, the automatic segmentation algorithm of SEPINRIA software [38] based on T1, T2, DP and Flair contrast images. Second, a manual correction of the lesion mask was done by a neurologist. The lesion load value (%) was obtained by dividing the lesion mask volume by the whole brain volume.

Region of Interest Approach

All image post-processing was performed on a Windows PC workstation independent of the imager. Post-processing of DTI data was performed using MedINRIA software [39]. After tensor calculation, maps of FA, ADC and $\lambda 1$, $\lambda 2$ and $\lambda 3$ were measured and derived on a pixel by pixel basis. Corpus callosum (CC) and centrum semioval (CSO) regions of interest were delimited on 5 consecutive 2.5 mm^3 thick slices of the FA maps (Figure 2). Histograms of ROIs values were fitted to provide peak position values.

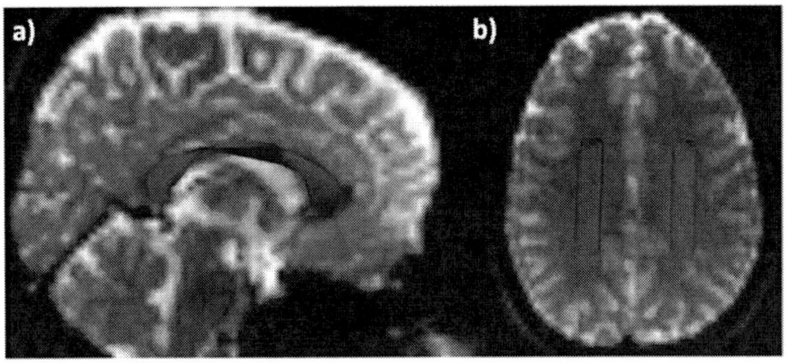

Figure 2. Corpus callosum (a) and Centrum semioval (b) regions of interest shown on diffusion images (b0).

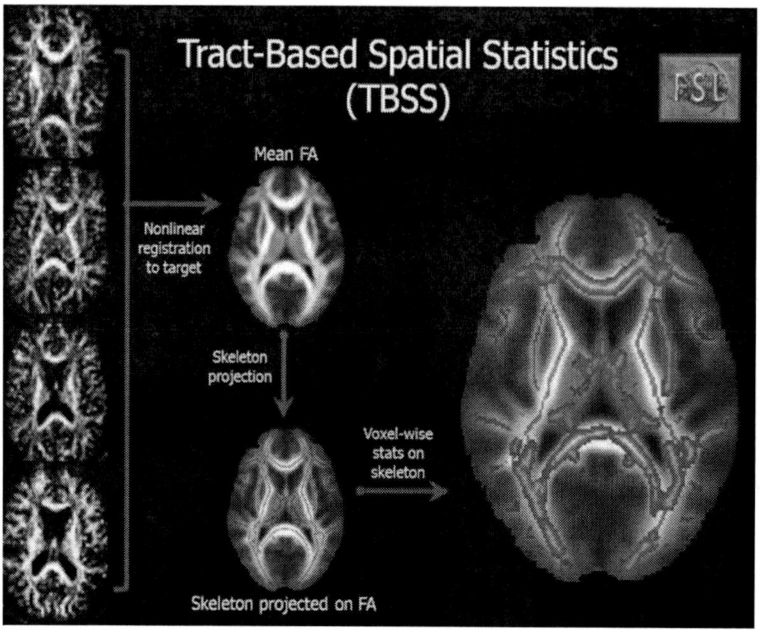

Figure 3. TBSS analysis pipeline.

TBSS Analysis

Post-processing of diffusion tensor data with TBSS was performed using FSL [36]. An eddy current correction using the FMRIB's Diffusion Toolbox (FDT) was applied followed by the extraction of non-brain voxels using the Brain Extraction Tool with a factor of 0.35. FA maps were then generated using FDT module. TBSS analysis consisted first in creating a mean skeleton from all patients and control subjects FA images by using an initial approximate nonlinear registration. Then, FA images of each subject are projected onto the skeleton by filling it with FA values from the nearest relevant tract centre (Figure 3).

Statistical Analysis

Statistical analysis of the ROIs DTI values was performed using Data Analysis and Statistical Software (STATA, Version 9.2, StataCorp, Texas, USA). Diffusivity values were compared between patients and controls using a One-Way ANOVA test. Bonferroni correction was used to perform post-hoc multiple comparisons. Spearman correlation test was applied to assess the relationship between diffusion metrics and lesion load and EDSS values. Correlations were not corrected for multiple comparisons. Cross-subject voxel-wise permutation based statistical TBSS analysis was performed using "randomise" module of FSL in between groups of patients and controls to produce maps of altered FA. Results were considered significant for a p value inferior to 0.05.

Results

ROI Measures

DTI-derived parameters measured from the CC and the CSO regions showed significant alterations in MS patients with different clinical forms (Table 2). Increases of both axial and radial diffusivity values, with a greater magnitude in the radial relative to the axial component, resulted in a highly significant increase in diffusivity and a significant reduction in anisotropy values. When comparing SP to RR patients, FA values were significantly lower (CC $p<0.001$; CSO $p<0.01$) while MD (CC $p<0.001$; CSO $p<0.01$), λa (CC $p<0.05$; CSO $p<0.05$) and λr (CC $p<0.001$; CSO $p<0.001$) values were higher in SP patients. In contrast, no significant changes were detected between PP and RR patients except in the CC where FA was significantly decreased ($p<0.05$) and λr increased ($p<0.05$).

Correlation with T2-LL and EDSS

RR and SP patients DTI values obtained from the CC and the CSO regions showed significant correlations with T2-LL as shown in Table 3 while no relation was found in PP patients (Figure 4).

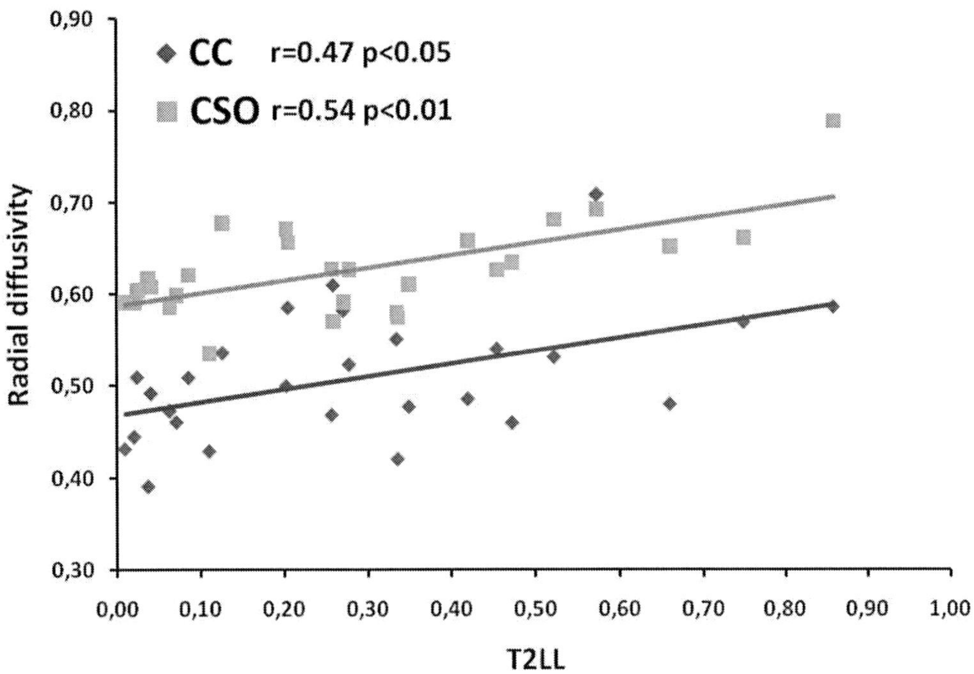

Figure 4. Correlation between the radial diffusivity measured in the corpus callosum (CC) and the centrum semioval (CSO) regions and the lesion load obtained by T2-hyperintensities volume measurement.

Table 2. Diffusion measures in the CC and the CSO regions

		Controls	RR	SP	PP
CC	FA	0.684 (0.020)	0.646 (0.038)**	0.582 (0.053)***	0.611 (0.044)***
	MD	0.782 (0.037)	0.879 (0.065)***	0.990 (0.117)***	0.940 (0.098)***
	λa	1.514 (0.060)	1.628 (0.071)***	1.702 (0.124)***	1.664 (0.106)***
	λr	0.418 (0.033)	0.509 (0.069)***	0.640 (0.124)***	0.584 (0.099)***
CSO	FA	0.400 (0.024)	0.378 (0.030)*	0.350 (0.034)***	0.368 (0.032)**
	MD	0.711 (0.027)	0.790 (0.048)***	0.858 (0.100)***	0.822 (0.087)***
	λa	1.031 (0.036)	1.117 (0.052)***	1.174 (0.100)***	1.150 (0.096)***
	λr	0.552 (0.028)	0.627 (0.050)***	0.700 (0.101)***	0.658 (0.085)***

Results are presented as mean (SD) (*p<0.05; **p<0.01; ***p<0.001) CC: corpus callosum; CSO: centrum semioval; FA: fractional anisotropy; MD: mean diffusivity; λa: axial diffusivity; λr: radial diffusivity; RR: relapsing remitting; SP: secondary progressive; PP: primary progressive.

No correlation were found with the EDSS scores when considering patients seperatly but when grouping them in one group of MS patients significant correlations were found between CC and CSO diffusivity measures (CC: FA: -0.28*; MD: r=0.27*; λr: 0.32**; CSO: FA: -0.32**; λr: 0.27*).

Results are presented as correlation coefficients (*p<0.05; **p<0.01; ***p<0.001) CC: corpus callosum; CSO: centrum semioval; FA: fractional anisotropy; MD: mean diffusivity; λa: axial diffusivity; λr: radial diffusivity; RR: relapsing remitting; SP: secondary progressive; PP: primary progressive.

TBSS Analysis

TBSS analysis showed FA reductions in different brain regions of MS patients (RR, SP and PP) compared with control subjects as reported in Figure 4. These results summarized in Table 4. RR patients present greater decreases of FA in the left hemisphere compared to the right hemisphere. This left-right difference disappears in the advanced form SP. When comparing RR to SP patients, significant FA differences were found in upper and inferior longitudinal fascicle, inferior fronto-occipital fascicle, cortico-spinal and uncinate tracts, thalamic radiations, internal and external capsules, corpus callosum and cingulum. Similarly, when comparing RR and PP patients (Table 4 and Figure5), FA decreases were especially found in the external capsule, corpus callosum and superior longitudinal fasciculus and inferior fronto-occipital fasciculus. In contrast, no significant difference appeared when comparing the SP and PP patients.

Table 3. Correlation results between DTI measures in the CC and the CSO regions and T2-LL

	CC				CSO			
	FA	MD	λa	λr	FA	MD	λa	λr
RR	-0.43 *	0.52**	0.51**	0.47*	-	0.63***	0.64***	0.53**
SP	-0.41*	0.52**	0.47*	0.42*	-0.41*	0.53**	0.54**	0.56**

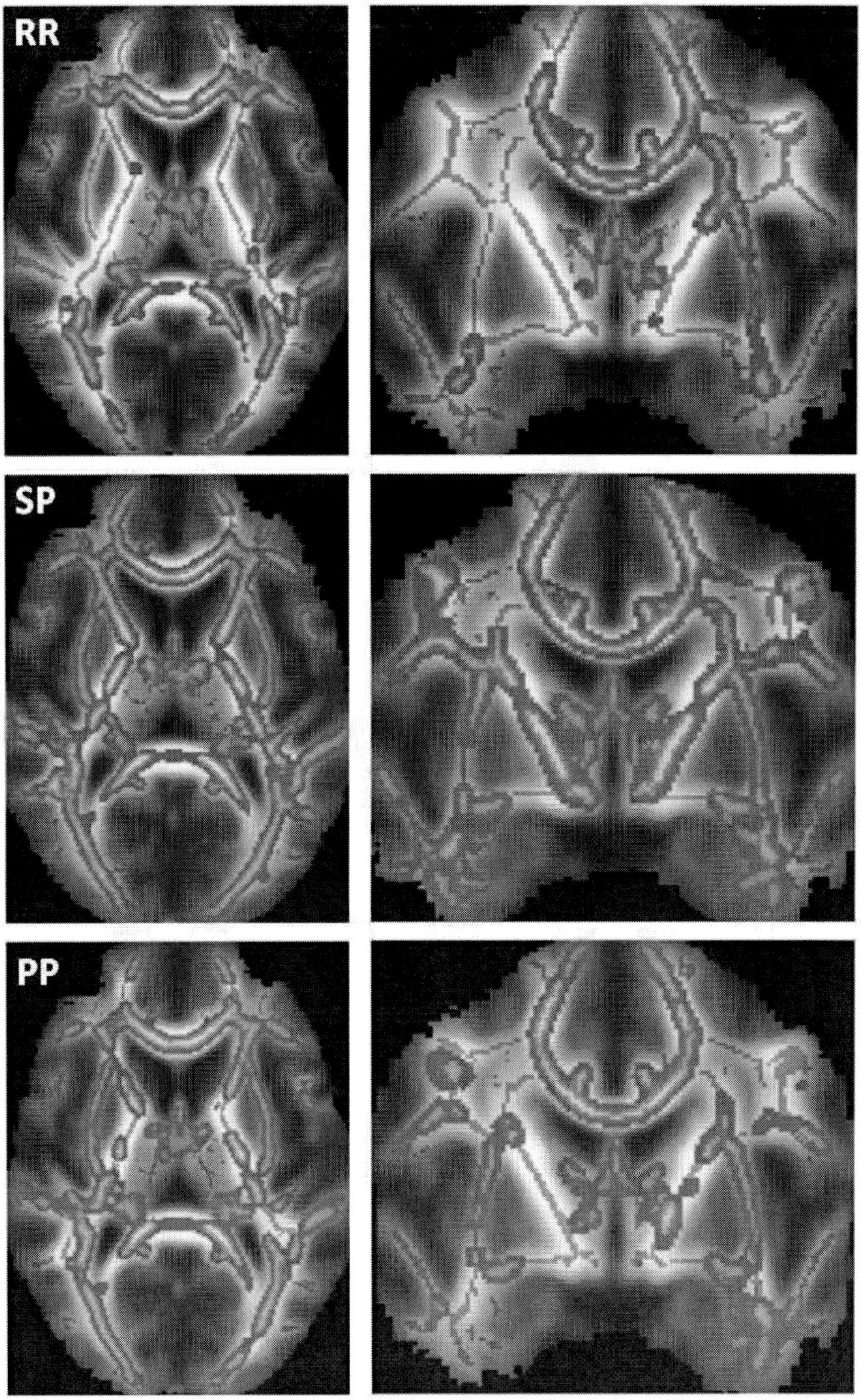

Figure 5. TBSS analysis of different clinical forms of MS patients including RR, SP, and PP compared to control subjects. Regions with significant FA reduction are shown in red.

Table 4. Decreased FA regions obtained by TBSS analysis in MS patients

Decreased FA Regions	RR *vs* C	SP *vs* C	PP *vs* C	SP *vs* RR	PP *vs* RR
Inferior longitudinal fasciculus L&R	$p<0.01$	$p<0.01$	$p<0.01$	$p<0.01$	$p<0.05$
Superior longitudinal fasciculus L	$p<0.01$	$p<0.01$	$p<0.01$	$p<0.01$	-
Superior longitudinal fasciculus R	-	$p<0.01$	$p<0.01$	$p<0.01$	$p<0.05$
Inferior fronto-occipital fasciculus L&R	$p<0.01$	$p<0.01$	$p<0.01$	$p<0.01$	$p<0.05$
Anterior thalamic radiation L	$p<0.01$	$p<0.01$	$p<0.01$	$p<0.01$	-
Anterior thalamic radiation R	$p<0.01$	$p<0.01$	$p<0.01$	$p<0.01$	$p<0.05$
Corticospinal tract L	$p<0.01$	$p<0.01$	$p<0.01$	$p<0.01$	$p<0.05$
Corticospinal tract R	-	$p<0.01$	$p<0.01$	$p<0.01$	$p<0.05$
Anterior limb of the internal capsule L&R	$p<0.01$	$p<0.01$	$p<0.01$	$p<0.01$	-
Posterior limb of the internal capsule L	-	$p<0.01$	$p<0.01$	$p<0.01$	-
Posterior limb of the internal capsule R	-	$p<0.01$	-	$p<0.01$	-
External capsule L	$p<0.01$	$p<0.01$	$p<0.01$	$P<0.01$	$p<0.05$
External capsule R	-	$p<0.01$	$p<0.01$	$P<0.01$	$p<0.05$
Corpus callosum genu	$p<0.01$	$p<0.01$	$p<0.01$	$P<0.01$	-
Corpus callosum body	$p<0.01$	$p<0.01$	$p<0.01$	$P<0.01$	$p<0.05$
Corpus callosum splenium	$p<0.01$	$p<0.01$	$p<0.01$	$P<0.01$	$p<0.05$
Forceps Minor	$p<0.01$	$p<0.01$	$p<0.01$	$P<0.01$	-
Forceps Major	$p<0.01$	$p<0.01$	$p<0.01$	$P<0.01$	$p<0.05$
Cingulum L&R	$p<0.01$	$p<0.01$	$p<0.01$	$P<0.01$	-
Uncinate fasciculus L&R	-	$p<0.01$	$p<0.01$	$P<0.01$	-

L: left; R: right; C: controls; RR: relapsing remitting; SP: secondary progressive; PP: primary progressive.

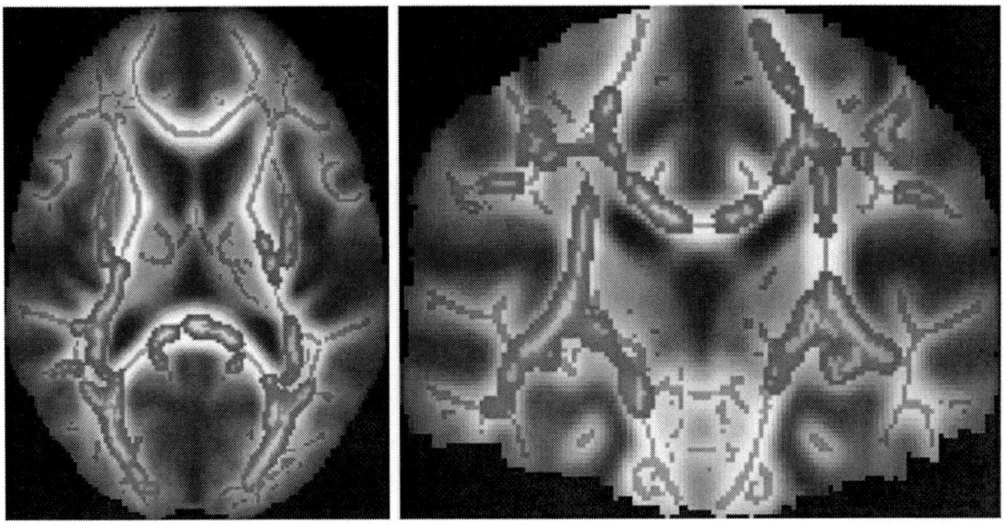

Figure 6. WM regions (red) of significant FA differences analyzed by TBSS between RR and PP patients are shown on axial (left) and coronal (right) views.

Discussion

In this study, we used two regional approaches to investigate the contribution of WM microstructure, measured by DTI, to the pathological processes of MS. On one hand, the ROI approach allowed us to determine the diffusivity values in two regions of WM, namely the corpus callosum and the central semioval regions. The quantification of DTI metrics demonstrated significant increases of MD, λa, and λr, and a decrease of FA in MS patients of any clinical form compared to control subjects. Moreover, these alterations were significantly greater in progressive forms compared to RR patients. These findings are in agreement with previous studies demonstrating that both CC and CSO are involved in MS disease [40].

These quantitative findings confirmed that the corpus callosum is early damaged in MS. The lesion load and the early atrophy measures are concordant with our results of correlation between the lesion load and the degree of DTI changes in RR and SP patients. The lack of correlation in PP patients suggest that microstructural alterations observed by DTI may be due to axonal degeneration induced by distal lesions instead of inflammatory attacks that are less frequent in PP patients [41]. Because the corpus callosum represents the largest WM fibre tract connecting both hemispheres and subcortical GM structures, local injury to the CC should lead to severe effects on brain functions as compared to CSO regions. This hypothesis is concordant with the modest correlation observed between DTI measures and EDSS in CC but not in CSO. However, the corpus callosum is a well organized and densely packed fibre structure that may be able to compensate local axonal damages by using other neural networks, explaining that damages remained subclinical. Nevertheless, DTI measurements in the corpus callosum may potentially constitute a sensitive marker of early microstructural alterations in CIS patients.

DTI abnormalities measured in the CSO regions suggested the presence of microscopic pathology beyond the sensitivity of conventional MRI. These findings are in agreement with previous studies demonstrating that DTI changes are widespread in NAWM but tend to be more severe in lesions and in periplaque regions [34]. Our results support this previous report as confirmed by the correlation observed between DTI values and lesion load. If all diffusion-derived parameters showed significant changes, radial diffusivity demonstrated the best sensitivity to reflect alterations in any clinical form, particularly in the primary RR form. In agreement with previous studies [35], these findings suggested that monitoring the tensor eigenvalues (axial and radial diffusivities) can provide better insights on various pathological processes. As reported in animal models of MS [42], the observation of greater increase in λr than in λa, leading to a significant decrease of anisotropy, may identify the occurrence of a primary myelin breakdown [36]followed by a secondary axonal damage [26, 43]. The exact pathological correlations with these changes of DTI values in WM are still not fully understood, although they are probably related to discrete inflammatory and demyelinating processes. Also, Wallerian degeneration may occur along the fiber pathway due to distant lesions [44] as suggested by the significant correlation found between lesion load and both axial and radial diffusivities.

If the ROI approach is well suited for an accurate analysis of a complete structure such as the corpus callosum, the reproducibility of ROI positioning between different study subjects is a source of error in the measurements. Furthermore, the selection of a large ROI such as the CSO which includes a mixture of NAWM and lesions induces bias in results interpretation. In contrast, the TBSS method based on a voxelwise analysis of WM fibre tracts is not affected by these disadvantages.

Interestingly, this TBSS study of different clinical forms demonstrated the increasing extent of microstructural alterations with the severity of the disease. In agreement with our ROI analysis of the CC and the CSO regions, FA was found to be abnormal in these regions of RR patients. These findings confirmed that these regions, particularly of the left hemisphere, are early altered by the disease. From the different regions reported in Table 4, the structure being most affected is the corpus callosum where the diffusivity is increased in all parts including genu, body and splenium. Along with the CC, the main interhemispheric connection, the major and minor forceps and the fornices were also subject to significant reductions of FA. Local transection of these fibre tracts could cause numerous cognitive deficits. In contrast, RR patients presenting less FA alterations suggest that they can compensate for the damage by functional reorganization [45-46].

Another major interconnecting tract, namely the inferior longitudinal fasciculus connects the occipital lobe with the parahippocampal gyrus and the lateral temporal lobe [47]. This network is known to have a major role in the visual memory of scenes, places recognition, as well as their emotional content [48]. Unfortunately, our patients did not perform any neuropsychological tests of visual memory that could provide information on the functional consequences of these damages. The left superior longitudinal fascicle (SLF) was also significantly altered as evidenced by the changes in anisotropy and diffusivity. As part of the default network evidenced by resting state functional MRI [49], the SLF connects the frontal and prefrontal regions with the parietal lobe. These bundles include also the arcuate fasciculus which connects the two language regions, namely Broca and Wernicke. Again, the lack of major language deficit, particularly in RR patients, suggests that these diffusivity changes may reflect preferentially local myelin injuries whose functional consequences remained subclinical.

Conclusion

These DTI measurements, analyzed either by a ROI quantification approach or a voxelwise statistical approach, demonstrated significant changes in MS patients of any clinical form. These findings confirmed that DTI is a very sensitive tool to detect early microscopic alterations in WM pathologies. Compared to the traditional ROI measures, TBSS provided a great advantage of an objective and statistical approach, and thus became a sensitive tool to compare groups of patients and subjects. However, the relation between these diffusivity markers and the underlying histopathological processes remains unknown. Further, the low spatial resolution of DTI associated with the complexity of modelling crossing fibres requires interpreting these data with caution. Thus, more developments are needed combining histopathology measures and improved DTI techniques to better understand these findings. Nevertheless, TBSS analysis of DTI can constitute a new input to investigate structural connectivity in conjunction with functional MRI and better understand the relationship between the neural substrate and the cognitive changes in MS.

Acknowledgments

This research was sponsored by the French government grant "PHRC 2004" and the Région Rhône-Alpes "Cluster11". The authors would like to express their gratitude to the staff of "CERMEP-Imagerie du Vivant" for their assistance in the acquisition of the data.

References

[1] McAlpine, D., & Compston, N. (1952). Some aspects of the natural history of disseminated sclerosis. *The Quarterly Journal of Medecine* , 21 (82), 135-167.

[2] Charcot, J. (1868). Histologie de la sclérose en plaques. *Gas Hop (Paris)* , 141, 554-558.

[3] McDonald, W., Compston, A., Edan, G., Goodkin, D., Hartung, H., Lublin, F., et al. (2001). Recommended diagnostic criteria for multiple sclerosis: guidelines from the international panel on the diagnosis of multiple sclerosis. *Annals of Neurology* , 50, 121-127.

[4] Fisniku, L.K., Brex, P.A., Altmann, D.R., Miszkiel, K.A., Benton, C.E., Lanyon, R., et al. (2008). Disability and T2 MRI lesions: a 20-year follow-up of patients with relapse onset of multiple sclerosis. *Brain* , 131(Pt 3), 808-817.

[5] De Groot, C.J., Bergers, E., Kamphorst, W., Ravid, R., Polman, C.H., Barkhof, F., et al. (2001). Post-mortem MRI-guided sampling of multiple sclerosis brain lesions: increased yield of active demyelinating and (p) reactive lesions. *Brain* , 124(Pt 8), 1635-1645.

[6] Moore, G.R., Leung, E., MacKay, A.L., Vavasour, I.M., Whittall, K.P., Cover, K.S., et al. (2000). A pathology-MRI study of the short-T2 component in formalin-fixed multiple sclerosis brain. Neurology , 55(10), 1506-1510.

[7] Bitsch, A., Kuhlmann, C., Stadelmann, C., Lassman, H., Lucchinetti, C., & Bruck, W. (2001). A longitudinal MRI study of histopathologically defined hypointense multiple sclerosis lesions. *Annals of Neurology , 49*, 793-796.

[8] Lumsden, C. (1970). The neuropathology of multiple sclerosis. Dans P. Vinken, & G. Bruyn, *Handbook of clinical neurology. Volume 9. Multiple sclerosis and other demyelinationg diseases* (pp. 217-309). New York: American Elsevier.

[9] Peterson, J., Bo, L., Mork, S., Chang, A., & Trapp, B. (2001). Transected neurites, apoptotic neurons, and reduced inflammation in cortical multiple sclerosis lesions. *Annals of Neurology , 50*, 389-400.

[10] Dawson, J. (1916). The histology of multiple sclerosis. *Trans R Soc (Ebind) , 50*, 517-740.

[11] Brownell, B., & Hughes, J.T. (1962). The distribution of plaques in the cerebrum in multiple sclerosis. *J. Neurol. Neurosurg. Psychiatry* , 25, 315-320.

[12] Kidd, D., Barkhof, F., McConnell, R., Algra, P., Allen, I., & Revesz, T. (1999). Cortical lesions in multiple sclerosis. *Brain , 122* (1), 17-26.

[13] Barkhof, F. (2002). The clinico-radiological paradox in multiple sclerosis revisited. *Current Opinion in Neurology , 15* (3), 239-245.

[14] Stejskal, E., & Tanner, J. (1965). Spin diffusion measurements: spin echoes in the presence of time-dependent field gradient. *The Journal of Chemical Physics , 42* (1), 288-292.

[15] Taylor, D., & Bushell, M. (1985). The spatial mapping of translational diffusion coefficients by the NMR imaging technique. *Physics in Medicine and Biology , 30* (4), 345-349.

[16] Le Bihan, D., & Breton, E. (1985). Imagerie de diffusion in vivo par résonance magnétique nucléaire. *Comptes Rendus de l'Académie des Sciences Paris , 301*, 1109-1112.

[17] Moseley, M., Cohen, Y., Kucharaczyj, M., Minotorovitch, J., Asgari, H., Wendland, M., et al. (1990). Diffusion-Weighted MR imaging of anisotropic water diffusion in cat central nervous system. *Radiology , 176*, 439-445.

[18] Moseley, M.E., Butts, K., Yenari, M.A., Marks, M., & de Crespigny, A. (1995). Clinical aspects of DWI. *NMR Biomed.* , 8(7-8), 387-396.

[19] Douek, P., Turner, R., Pekar, J., Patronas, N., & Le Bihan, D. (1991). MR color mapping of myelin fiber orientation. *Journal of Computer Assisted Tomography , 15* (6), 923-929.

[20] Basser, P., Mattiello J., & Le Bihan D. (1994). MR diffusion tensor spectoscopy and imaging. *Biophysical Journal.,* 66(1), 259-267.

[21] Westin, C., Maier, S., Mamata, H., Nabavi, A., Jolesz, F., & Kikinis, R. (2002). Processing and visualisation for diffusion tensor MRI. *Medical image analysis , 6*, 93-108.

[22] Pierpaoli, P., & Basser, P. (1996). Toward a quantitative assessment of diffusion anisotropy. *Magnetic Resonance in Medicine , 36*, 893-906.

[23] Peled, S., Gudbjartsson, H., Westin, C., Kikins, R., & Jolesz, F. (1998). Magnetic resonance imaging shows orientation and asymmetry of white matter fiber tracts. *Brain Research , 780*, 27-33.

[24] Tuch, D.S., Reese, T.G., Wiegell, M.R., Makris, N., Belliveau, J.W., & Wedeen, V.J. (2002). High angular resolution diffusion imaging reveals intravoxel white matter fiber heterogeneity. *Magn Reson Med.* , 48(4), 577-582.

[25] Wedeen, V.J., Wang, R.P., Schmahmann, J.D., Benner, T., Tseng, W.Y., Dai, G., et al. (2008). Diffusion spectrum magnetic resonance imaging (DSI) tractography of crossing fibers. *Neuroimage* , 41(4), 1267-1277.

[26] Rovaris, M., Gass, A., Bammer, R., Hickman, S., Ciccarelli, O., Miller, D., et al. (2005). Diffusion MRI in multiple sclerosis. *Neurology , 65*, 1526-1532.

[27] Goldberg-Zimring, D., Mewes, A., Maddah, M., & Warfield, S. (2005). Diffusion tensor magnetic resonance imaging in multiple sclerosis. *Journal of Neuroimaging , 15* (4 Suppl), 68S-81S.

[28] Ciccarelli, O., Werring, D., Barker, G., Griffin, C., Wheeler-Kingshott, C., Miller, D., et al. (2003). A study of the mechanisms of normal-appearing white matter damage in multiple sclerosis using diffusion tensor imaging--evidence of Wallerian degeneration. *Journal of Neurology , 250* (3), 287-292.

[29] Castriota-Scanderberg, A., Fasano, F., Hagberg, G., Nocentini, U., Filippi, M., & Caltagirone, C. (2003). Coefficient D(av) is more sensitive than fractional anisotropy in monitoring progression of irreversible tissue damage in focal nonactive multiple sclerosis lesions. *AJNR American Journal of Neuroradiology , 24* (4), 663-670.

[30] Werring, D., Brassat, D., Droogan, A., Clark, C., Symms, M., Barker, G., et al. (2000). The pathogenesis of lesions and normal-appearing white matter changes in multiple sclerosis: a serial diffusion MRI study. *Brain , 123* (Pt8), 1667-1676.

[31] Roychowdhury, S., Maldjian, J., & Grossman, R. (2000). Multiple sclerosis: comparison of trace apparent diffusion coefficients with MR enhancement pattern of lesions. *AJNR American Journal of Neuroradiology , 21* (5), 869-874.

[32] Cercignani, M., Inglese, M., Pagani, E., Comi, G., & Filippi, M. (2001). Mean diffusivity and fractional anisotropy histograms of patients with multiple sclerosis. *AJNR American Journal of Neuroradiology , 22*, 952-958.

[33] Ge, Y., Law, M., & Grossman, R. (2005). Applications of diffusion tensor MR imaging in multiple sclerosis. *Annals of the New York Academy of Sciences , 1064*, 202-219.

[34] Guo, A., MacFall, J., & Provenzale, J. (2002). Multiple sclerosis: diffusion tensor MR imaging for evaluation of normal-appearing white matter. *Radiology , 222*, 729-736.

[35] Lowe, M., Horenstein, C., Hirsch, J., Marrie, R., Stone, L., Bhattacharyya, P., et al. (2006). Functional pathway-defined MRI diffusion measures reveal increased transverse diffusivity of water in multiple sclerosis. *Neuroimage , 32* (3), 1127-1133.

[36] Smith, S., Jenkinson, M., Johansen-Berg, H., Rueckert, D., Nichols, T., Mackay, C., et al. (2006). Tract-based spatial statistics: Voxelwise analysis of multi-subject diffusion data. *Neuroimage , 31*, 1487-1505.

[37] Roosendaal, S.D., Geurts, J.J., Vrenken, H., Hulst, H.E., Cover, K.S., Castelijns, J.A., et al. (2009). Regional DTI differences in multiple sclerosis patients. *Neuroimage ,* 44(4), 1397-1403.

[38] Souplet, J.C. Évaluation de l'atrophie et de la charge lésionnelle sur des séquences IRM de patients atteints de sclérose en plaques. PhD Thesis Université de Nice Sophia-Antipolis, January 2009.

[39] Toussaint, N., Souplet, J., & Fillard, P. (2007). MedINRIA: Medical image navigation and research tool by INRIA. Brisbane, Australia.

[40] Ge, Y., Law, M., Johnson, G., Herbert, J., Babb, J., Mannon, L., et al. (2004). Preferential occult injury of corpus callosum in multiple sclerosis measured by diffusion tensor imaging. *Journal of Magnetic Resonance Imaging , 20* (1), 1-7.

[41] Miller, D.H., & Leary, S.M. (2007).Primary-progressive multiple sclerosis. *Lancet Neurol.* , 6, 903-912.

[42] Song, S., Yoshino, J., Le, T., Lin, S., Sun, S., Cross, A., et al. (2005). Demyelination increases radial diffusivity in corpus callosum of mouse brain. *Neuroimage , 26* (1), 132-140.

[43] Pierpaoli, C., Barnett, A., Pajejevic, S., Chen, R., Penix, L., Virta, A., et al. (2001). Water diffusion changes in Wallerian degeneration and their dependence on white matter architecture. *Neuroimage , 13* (6Pt1), 1174-1185.

[44] De Stefano, N., Iannucci, G., Sormani, M., Guidi, L., Bartolozzi, M., Comi, G., et al. (2002). MR correlates of cerebral atrophy in patients with multiple sclerosis. *Journal of Neurology , 249* (8), 1072-1077.

[45] Ciccarelli, O., Toosy, A.T., Marsden, J.F., Wheeler-Kingshott, C.M., Miller, D.H., Matthews, P.M., et L. (2006). Functional response to active and passive ankle movements with clinical correlations in patients with primary progressive multiple sclerosis. *J Neurol.* , 253(7), 882-891.

[46] Mainero, C., Caramia, F., Pozzilli, C., Pisani, A., Pestalozza, I., Borriello, G.,et al. (2004). fMRI evidence of brain reorganization during attention and memory tasks in multiple sclerosis. *Neuroimage* , 21(3), 858-867.

[47] Catani, M., Jones, D., Donato, R., & Flytche, D. (2003). Occipito-temporal connections in the human brain. *Brain , 126*, 2093-2107.

[48] Murty, V.P., Ritchey, M., Adcock, R.A., & Labar,K.S. (2011). Reprint of: fMRI studies of successful emotional memory encoding: A quantitative meta-analysis. *Neuropsychologia* , 49(4), 695-705.

[49] Liu, Y., Liang, P., Duan, Y., Jia, X., Yu, C., Zhang, M., et al. (2011). Brain plasticity in relapsing-remitting multiple sclerosis: Evidence from resting-state fMRI. *J Neurol Sci.* [Epub ahead of print]

In: Multiple Sclerosis
Editor: E. Scholz and C. Müller, pp. 131-142
ISBN 978-1-61324-848-5

Chapter VII

Immunoglobulin Free Light Chains in the Diagnosis of Multiple Sclerosis

Batia Kaplan[1,*], ***Sizilia Golderman***[1] ***and Ben-Ami Sela***[2,3]
[1]Heller Institute of Medical Research, Sheba Medical Center, Tel-Hashomer, Israel
[2]Institute of Chemical Pathology, Sheba Medical Center, Tel-Hashomer, Israel
[3]Sackler School of Medicine, Tel-Aviv University, Tel-Aviv, Israel

Abstract

The diagnosis of multiple sclerosis (MS) is based on clinical criteria, magnetic resonance imaging (MRI) data and laboratory findings. The latter include information obtainable from analysis of cerebrospinal fluid (CSF) where demonstration of oligoclonal immunoglobulin G (IgG) bands (OCB) indicates an intrathecal production of IgGs and supports diagnosis of MS. One of the major disadvantages of this commonly used test is that OCBs might be detected in other inflammatory and infectious diseases of the central nervous system. Thus, search for novel technologies and new MS-specific markers is of diagnostic value.

This review highlights the potential importance of Ig free light chains (FLCs) as novel diagnostic markers for MS. Different methods applied to analyze FLCs in the CSF of MS patients are described. These include immunochemical methods based on electrophoretic techniques, as well as radioimmunoassay and nephelometric immunoassay. Application of these methods brought valuable information with regard to the characteristic features of FLCs in MS: κ and λ level, their oligoclonality and monomer-dimer patterns. In this review, the advantages and disadvantages of the reported methods are discussed with respect to their specificity, sensitivity, complexity and availability. While none of the reported methods is perfect, many of them may complement each other by providing a more comprehensive characterization of FLCs in MS. Considering the heterogeneous nature of MS, such information may assist in further

* Correspondence to: Batia Kaplan, PhD. Heller Institute of Medical Research, Sheba Medical Center, Tel-Hashomer 52621, Israel. Phone: +972-3-530-3363; E-mail: batiakaplan@gmail.com.

studies aimed to establish new laboratory markers for different forms and stages of this disease.

Introduction

Multiple sclerosis (MS) is a central nervous system (CNS)-specific, putatively autoimmune disease that triggers inflammation in the brain and spinal cord and results in demyelination, axonal damage and neuronal loss. As in other chronic inflammatory diseases, the CNS of patients with multiple sclerosis shows infiltration of activated T cells and macrophages, dendritic cells, B cells and plasma cells. This implies potential roles for both cellular and humoral immune responses and the engagement of different immunopathological effector mechanisms yielding CNS tissue destruction [1]. The diagnosis for MS is based on clinical criteria, magnetic resonance imaging (MRI) data and laboratory findings [2]. The latter include information obtainable from analysis of cerebrospinal fluid (CSF) where demonstration of oligoclonal immunoglobulin G (IgG) bands (OCBs) indicates an intrathecal production of Igs and supports the diagnosis of MS.

Although demonstration of OCBs in CSF is a commonly accepted test in MS management, OCBs might be detected in other inflammatory and infectious CNS diseases [3]. Another disadvantage of the OCB test is that this technique is qualitative and highly depends on skills and experience of laboratory personnel. Problems might also arise with the interpretation of a single weak band, and additional techniques might be crucial to obtain a more conclusive diagnosis. In this respect, development of novel laboratory techniques and the search for new reliable MS-specific markers remains of considerable diagnostic importance for MS.

The potential importance of immunoglobulin free light chains (FLCs) in the diagnosis of MS was first described in the late 70s. Early immunochemical methods were mainly based on electrophoretic techniques, such as immunoelectrophoresis [4, 5], sodium dodecyl sulfate polyacrylamide gel electrophoresis (SDS-PAGE) [6], agarose electrophoresis or isoelectrofocusing [7-9]. These studies demonstrated increased levels of FLCs in the CSF of MS patients. The applied methods, however, were basically qualitative, their specificity in MS remains questionable, and they are not used for routine CSF analyses. For quantification of FLCs in CSF, radioimmunoassay [10, 11] and nephelometric immunoassay [12-14] were applied. Recently, the nephelometric FLC assay [15, 16] gained special attention in MS studies. In contrast to the OCB test, this FLC test is highly automated, it allows quantitative determination of FLCs, and demonstrates the significantly increased κ type FLC levels in MS. However, albeit the high sensitivity of the nephelometric FLC assay [12-14], its specificity was lower than that of the conventional OCB test [13, 14]. As a result, the OCB test still prevails as the most commonly used laboratory method to support the diagnosis of MS.

In a recent study in our laboratory we applied Western blot technique to analyze the monomer-dimer patterns of κ and λ type FLCs in patients with MS and other neurological diseases [17]. The combined use of the FLC indices accounting for monomeric and dimeric FLC-κ and λ levels and κ/λ ratio values in CSF and serum, was found to show some promising improvements in the diagnosis of MS.

This review is focused on FLC studies in MS including the issues of FLC production within CNS, the possible role of FLCs in MS pathogenesis and their diagnostic value. The importance of FLCs as a biomarker for MS is highlighted. Advantages and disadvantages of different methods for FLC analysis are discussed with respect to their utility as diagnostic tests for MS.

FLCs in Health and Disease

Human immunoglobulin (Ig) molecules consist of two identical heavy chains and two identical light chains. The latter exist as two isotypes, κ or λ, and they are covalently linked to heavy chains. Any given antibody molecule has either κ or λ-type light chain but not both. FLC-κ molecules (chromosome 2) are constructed from about forty functional Vκ gene segments, five Jκ gene segments and a single Cκ gene. FLC-λ molecules (chromosome 22) are constructed from approximately thirty Vλ gene segments, four pairs of functional Jλ gene segments and a Cλ gene. FLCs are incorporated into Ig molecules during B lymphocyte development and are expressed initially on the surface of pre B-cells. Production of FLCs occurs throughout the rest of B-cell development and in plasma cells, where the secretion is highest [16].

Normally, light chains are produced in excess over heavy chains. In a healthy state, the majority of light chains in the serum are bound to heavy chains, and the serum level of the secreted unbound light chains, i.e., so-called free light chains (FLCs), is low. FLCs can also be detected in urine, cerebrospinal fluid and synovial fluid, where the physiological levels of FLCs are also low. Under pathological conditions, however, production of FLCs might be abnormally high [16]). In monoclonal gammopathies, such as multiple myeloma, primary systemic amyloidosis (AL amyloidosis), and non-amyloid light chain deposition disease, the levels of monoclonal FLCs in the serum are significantly increased. Serum levels of polyclonal FLCs might be markedly elevated in some patients with inflammatory or autoimmune diseases associated with generalized increased B-cell activation, e.g., systemic lupus erithematosus, AIDS, and Sjogren's disease. In MS, because of the inflammation of CNS, synthesis of intrathecal FLCs leads to their accumulation in the CSF of the affected patients.

FLC molecules are usually monomers and dimers but higher polymeric forms might also exist [18-22]. Dimeric FLC are composed of two identical monomeric FLCs (either kappa or lambda) bound to each other by covalent or non-covalent links. λ FLCs have a stronger tendency to dimerization (and oligomerization) compared to that of κ FLCs [20, 21]. In the non-covalent dimerization of FLCs, the intermolecular electrostatic, hydrophobic and hydrogen bonds may play a role. Covalent binding of FLC monomers into dimers involves formation of an interchain disulfide bond between C-terminal FLC cysteins via oxidation of their thiol (SH) groups acting as electron donors. Formation of disulfide bonds occurs intracellulary and is catalyzed by a family of oxi-reductases. Activity of these enzymes depends on the environmental conditions within the cell, especially on redox potential [23, 24]. Under pathological conditions, however, shift in redox potential may occur thus affecting the subtle balance between monomeric and dimeric states. Alternatively, the peculiarities of FLC structure caused by somatic mutations or/and post-translational modifications might also affect formation of inter-molecular disulfide bonds [25]. Marked increase in the level of dimeric and multimeric FLC forms was demonstrated in the serum of patients with monoclonal gammopathies, such as multiple myeloma [22, 26] and AL amyloidosis [27]. Our recent study showed significant increase in the proportion of dimeric λ FLCs in the CSF of about 50% of the tested MS patients [17].

Intrathecal Production of FLCs and their Role in MS

Intrathecal antibody production and presence of oligoclonal IgGs in the CSF are the characteristic features of MS. Therefore, many studies are focused on the elucidation of mechanisms of B-cell trafficking, survival, and differentiation in the CNS leading to the intrathecal Ig synthesis. It was found that peripherally activated B-cells (plasmablasts) may be selectively recruited to MS brain where they differentiate into antibody producing cells. Alternatively, the circulating memory B-cells might enter the CNS and then expand and mature locally mimicking a germinal center reaction [28, 29]. The lymphoid follicle-like structures in the cerebral meninges were detected in about 40% of the secondary progressive MS cases [1]. These findings support the view that B-cell maturation can be sustained locally within the CNS and contribute to the establishment of a compartmentalized humoral immune response.

Intrathecal production of FLCs in MS usually occurs alongside production of intact IgGs. However, in some MS cases the abnormal increase in κ FLCs in CSF was observed without concomitant increase in IgG production [13, 30] and in the absence of oligoclonal IgG banding [17, 13, 31, 32]. These studies suggest that production of FLCs might be selectively increased as a result of an ongoing intrathecal humoral immune response [33].

Despite the considerable progress toward understanding the humoral immune response developing in the CNS of MS patients, it was not yet clarified whether the intrathecally produced antibodies are relevant to the pathology of this disease [34]. In respect to intrathecal FLCs, they have been long considered as the meaningless remnants of spillover in Ig production by B-cells [35]. However, the recently discovered ability of FLCs to sensitize mast cells shed new light on their potential role in immune responses. It was shown that κ FLCs induce mast cells degranulation and de novo synthesis and release of inflammatory mediators [33, 35, 36]. Significant elevation of the specific mast cell markers in the CSF of MS patients [35, 37, 38], increased number of mast cells in MS brain [35], together with increased CSF levels of FLC in this disease [12-14, 17], support the view that FLCs may play a role in the pathogenesis of MS [38]. However, many important questions must be answered before a role for FLCs in MS can be ascertained. It still remains unclear whether FLCs interact with mast cells, and if so, the elucidation of membrane receptor involved in FLC-mediated responses will become crucial [35]. Further studies are required to understand the mechanism of mast cell activation in MS.

Analysis of Intrathecal κ and λ FLCs in MS

FLCs were first detected in the CSF of MS patients by using single radial immunodiffusion [39, 40]. The following early studies were mainly based on agarose electrophoresis or isoelectrofocusing [7-9] and radioimmunoassay [10, 11]. In some studies the predominance of λ over κ-type FLCs was demonstrated [7, 41]. Other studies, however, showed the abnormally high CSF level of κ rather than λ-FLCs [10, 11]. Oligoclonality of both κ and λFLCs was revealed in most MS patients by employing an affinity mediated capillary blotting technique [9]. Similarly, isoelectrofocusing of CSF samples from 50 patients with definite MS diagnosis demonstrated oligoclonal banding of κ and λ FLCs in 92% and 86% MS cases, respectively [42]. However, since the increased κ and λ levels and the oligoclonality of FLCs were also observed in other non-MS neurological diseases, the utility of FLC testing in the diagnosis of MS is still questionable.

At present, due to the development of a highly automated nephelometrc FLC assay [16], there is a growing renewed interest in CSF FLCs as potential markers for MS [12-14, 43]. In contrast to the previously used electrophoresis-based immunochemical techniques, the nephelometric FLC assay allowed quantification of κ and λ FLCs. The developed method also made possible construction of FLC indices to account for the differences in FLC level in patient's CSF and serum (FLC CSF/serum ratio), and for the deterioration of blood-CSF-barrier (albumin CSF/serum ratio). Comparison of κ and λ FLC index values determined by this assay showed that κ-FLC index was more specifically related to MS comparing with λ-FLC index [13, 14]. In MS, the κ-FLC indices varied from 2 to 618, and were significantly higher as compared to those in other non-inflammatory CNS diseases (from 1 to 74) [13]. According to another report [14], κ-FLC indices ranged from 2.03 to 1514 in MS, whereas the highest κ-FLC index value in a control group was 6.18. Thus, the increased intrathecal production of κ type FLCs was considered as an important pathological feature characterizing MS.

Although high values of κ-FLCs values were typically found in MS patients, it remains uncertain whether the intrathecal κ level may serve as an independent diagnostic parameter. Both κ and λ may be significantly increased not only in MS but also in other non-MS inflammatory diseases [43]. Quantification of κ-FLCs in CSF by nephelometric assay showed high sensitivity in detecting MS, however, the specificity of this assay was lower than of the OCB test [14] and even lower than the IgG index [13]. Most probably, the increased κ-FLC values are suggestive of MS, hence this FLC parameter together with other laboratory data and clinical indications, should be taken into consideration in the diagnosis of MS.

The predictive value of FLC analysis remains unclear. Some studies pointed to the predictive values of FLC-κ levels in CSF for the progression on expanded disability status score (EDSS) in MS ([44, 45]. Other authors, however, found no relationship between FLC-κ index and duration of disease or MS progression evaluated by EDSS [13].

Although the utility of FLCs in the diagnosis of MS still raises many questions, there is no doubt that both thc clcctrophoretic techniques and the nephelometric assay mentioned above are useful to elucidate the distinct pathological features of immunoglobulin synthesis in this disease. In this respect, it is noteworthy that selection of the method for FLC analysis, as well as interpretation of the obtained data, should be done by taking into account the advantages and disadvantages of the used techniques. The electrophoresis-based techniques are usually qualitative, more laborious and less sensitive as compared to nephelometric FLC assay. However, these techniques are relatively inexpensive and could be easily applied in clinical laboratories. In contrast, the nephelometric assay is rapid, simple and allows quantitative determination of the FLC level. However, this assay requires special and expensive equipment which may not be available in clinical laboratories. Another limit of the nephelometric FLC assay is the overestimation of FLC values in samples containing high amounts of dimeric and multimeric forms of FLCs [46, 47], that may complicate the interpretation of the obtainable data.

Thus, it appears that there is no single perfect method of FLC analysis to diagnose MS. Comparison of data obtained by FLC analysis and by other laboratory tests (including oligoclonal IgG banding) seems to be important, whereas search for new diagnostic FLC tests remains to be challenging.

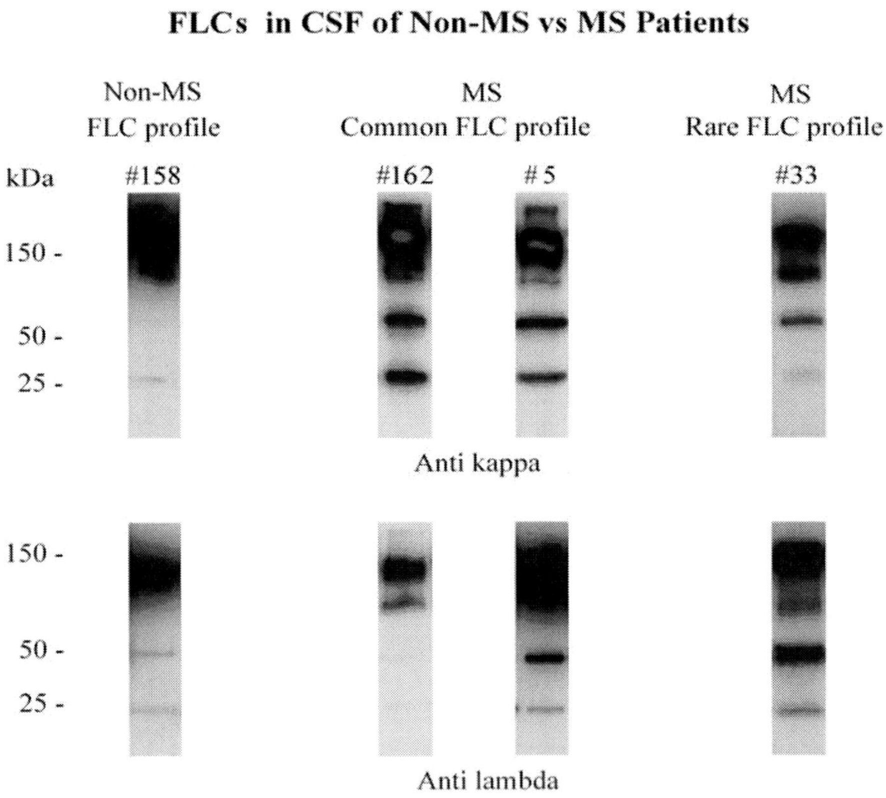

Figure 1. Western blot analysis of FLCs in the CSF of MS (cases #162, 5, 33) versus non-MS (case #158) patients. Samples were run by SDS-PAGE on 10-20% polyacrylamide gels under non-reducing conditions and immunostained using anti-κ and anti-λ antibodies. Typical examples of the common and rare FLC profiles in MS are displayed. The commonly observed FLC profile (#162 and 5) show the significantly increased levels of κ monomers and dimers, as well as the increase of κ /λ monomer ratios. The level of λ dimers is patient-specific. The rare MS profile (#33) is characterized by significantly elevated lambda dimers, whereas the levels of kappa and lambda monomers are law.

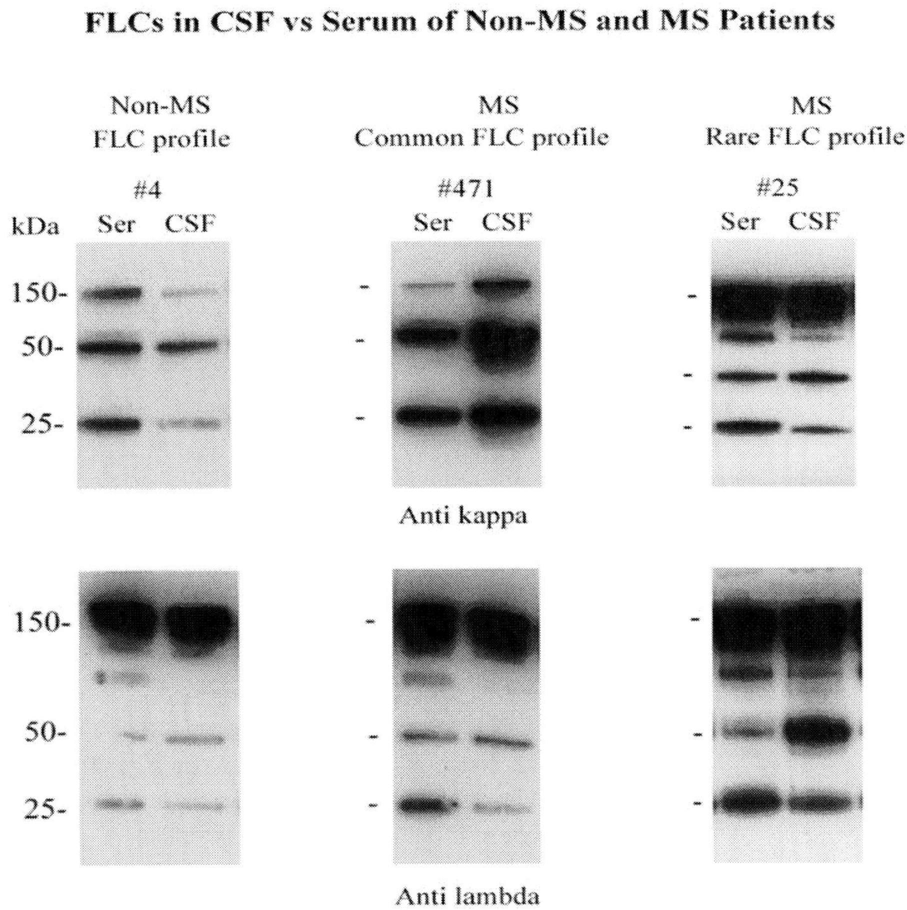

Figure 2. Western blot analysis of FLCs in the CSF versus serum of MS (cases #471 and 25) and non-MS (case #4) patients. Samples were run by SDS-PAGE on 10-20% polyacrylamide gels under non-reducing conditions and immunostained using anti-κ and anti-λ antibodies. Typical examples of FLC profiles in the CSF and serum of the same patients are displayed. In a common FLC profile observed in MS (#471), κ/λ monomer ratio in the CSF is high comparing to that in the serum. In the rare FLC profile (#25), λ dimer/monomer ratio is high in the CSF comparing with that in the serum. None of these FLC patterns in CSF versus serum is observed in the non-MS case (#4).

Analysis of Monomeric and Dimeric FLCs in MS

In our search for new diagnostic FLC parameters, we relied on our and findings of others, pointing to abnormal changes in the dimerization and polymerization of FLCs under certain pathological conditions, such as multiple myeloma, amyloidosis and non-amyloid light chain deposition disease [22, 25, 27, 48, 49]. Therefore, in contrast to the previously reported techniques used for FLC analysis, we evaluated the level of monomeric and covalently bound dimeric FLCs by employing the non-reducing SDS-PAGE coupled with immunoblotting [17]. In this report, data analysis was based on a quantitative evaluation of the intensity of immunoreactive bands of κ and λ monomers and dimers, as a measure of their levels in the CSF and serum. The intensity of the immunoreactive bands of the tested CSF samples was normalized with that of the positive control (MS) sample (ratio of the intensity of immunoreactive band in the control to that in the tested sample). Abnormally increased levels of monomeric and dimeric κ-FLC were observed in the MS group (18 patients with definite MS diagnosis and 3 MS/CIS patients) as compared to control group (n=8) and a large part of patients with other non-MS neurological diseases (20 out of 29). In contrast to κ-FLCs, the level of λ monomer in MS was low and comparable to that of the controls. The level of lambda dimer, however, varied within the MS group from normal to highly increased values. We found that κ but not λ level, as well as monomeric rather than dimeric κ/λ ratios are the preferable FLC parameters for differentiation between MS and non-MS patient groups. Three most informative diagnostic FLC indices were selected: a) CSF κ index accounting for monomer level (Test 1), b) CSF κ/λ monomer index (Test 2), c) ratio of κ/λ monomer intensity values in the serum to that in CSF (Test 3). Although each of these selected tests allowed the statistically significant differentiation between the MS and non-MS patient groups, none of these FLC indices taken separately was efficient enough to differentiate MS from other neurological diseases. However, the combined use of these FLC indices was highly effective for the diagnosis of MS. Mathematical multiplication of the above mentioned FLC index values was used to construct the Combined Test Index for monomers (CTIm). It allowed the determination of threshold value to efficiently differentiate MS from the non-MS cases. The developed FLC method demonstrated high specificity and sensitivity for MS as compared to the conventional OCB test applied for the same patients.

Our current examination of CSF samples was carried out with an extended number of patients with definite MS diagnosis (n=46). This study revealed some rare MS cases showing normal levels of κ and λ monomers, but the abnormally high level of λ dimers. Such pathological FLC pattern was not observed in the non-MS group (unpublished data). Taken together our reported data [17] and our new findings, we assume that the intrathecal FLCs in MS exhibit two different pathological profiles. In a common FLC profile (found in about 90% MS cases), significantly increased κ monomer and dimer levels are observed. In such cases, λ monomer level is close to that observed in the controls, while λ dimer level is patient-specific and varies from normal to high values. In a less frequent FLC MS profile (about 10%), the most prominent feature is the increase in λ dimer level; no significant increase was found in κ and λ type monomer level (Figure 1). Figure 2 demonstrates differences between the FLC profiles in CSF versus that in the serum of the same MS patient. In a common FLC profile observed in MS, κ/λ monomer ratio in the CSF is high in comparison to that in the serum. In the less frequent FLC profile, λ dimer/monomer ratio was high in the CSF comparing with that in the serum. Thus, for the quantitative assessment of the less frequent FLC profiles in MS, the following FLC indices was determined: CSF λ dimer level index (Test 4), CSF λ dimer/monomer ratio index (Test 5), and ratio of λ dimer/monomer value in the serum to that in the CSF (Test 6). We found that Combined Test Index for dimers (CTId) constructed using multiplication of Test 4, Test 5, and Test 6 values could be used as an additional test to diagnose MS. According to the results of our previous report [17] and those obtained by our presently conducted study, most MS patients show normal level of λ monomer but an abnormally high level of κ monomer and a CTIm value of less than 4 (common FLC profile in MS). In some less frequent MS cases, however, κ and λ monomer levels are close to normal, but λ dimers are significantly elevated and the CTId value is <0.007. Based on these criteria, analysis of 46 cases with definite MS and 37cases with other non-MS neurological diseases showed high specificity (95.7%) and sensitivity (95.6%) of the applied technique. Oligoclonality test applied for the same patients yielded a specificity of 80% and sensitivity of 85.1%. Thus, analysis of monomer-dimer profiles of κ and λ FLCs appears to be of promising diagnostic importance in MS.

Conclusions

Intrathecal production of FLCs is now regarded as an important part of humoral immune response developing in the CNS of MS patients. In this respect, detection and analysis of FLCs is of considerable interest, as it could contribute to the diagnosis of MS and may help to explore the possible link between FLC parameters and the form, stage and severity of MS disease. In most reports, importance of either κ-FLC level or FLC oligoclonality was highlighted as a characteristic feature of MS. However, the specificity of such tests based on a single FLC parameter was insufficient to differentiate MS from other neurological diseases. In our methodological approach, different FLC parameters were taken into consideration to support or exclude the diagnosis of MS. In contrast to the nephelometric FLC assay which allows an estimation of the total amount of all molecular forms of FLCs (monomers. dimers and multimers), our technique makes possible differential analysis of FLC monomers and covalently bound dimers. We revealed abnormalities of FLC dimerization in the CSF of MS patients, and this finding was taken into account when selecting the diagnostically useful markers for MS. The developed method showed high specificity and sensitivity as compared to the commonly used IgG oligoclonality test.

Although the reported methods of FLC analysis are different in their sensitivity and specificity, some of them may complement each other by providing a more comprehensive characterization of FLCs, for example, determination of oligoclonality of FLCs (by isoelectrofocusing or high resolution agarose gel electrophoresis), pI (isoelectrofocusing), concentration (nephelometry), monomer-dimer pattern (SDS-PAGE). Considering the heterogeneous nature of MS, such information may assist in the further studies aimed to establish new laboratory markers for different forms and stages of this disease.

References

[1] Magliozzi R, Howell O, Vora A, Serafini B, Nicholas R, Puopolo M, et al. Meningeal B-cell follicles in secondary progressive multiple sclerosis associate with early onset of disease and severe cortical pathology. *Brain* 2007;130:1089-104.

[2] Freedman MS, Thomson EJ, Deisenhammer F, Giovannoni G, Grimsley G, Keir G, et al. Recommended standard of cerebrospinal fluid analysis in the diagnosis of multiple sclerosis. A consensus statement. *Arch Neurol.* 2005;62:865-70.

[3] Jenkins MA, Cheng L, Ratnaike S. Multiple sclerosis: use of light-chain typing to assist diagnosis. *Ann Clin Biochem.* 2001;38:235-41.

[4] Vandvik B. Oligoclonal IgG and free light chains in the cerebrospinal fluid of patients with multiple sclerosis and infectious diseases of the central nervous system. *Scan J Immunol.* 1977;6: 913-22.

[5] Perini JM, Lebas J, Roussel P, Biserte G. Evidence for heterogeneous or incomplete immunoglobulins in oligoclonal CSF studied by electroimmunofixation. *Clin Chim Acta_1979*;96:205-14.

[6] Rudick RA, Peter DR, Bidlack JM, Knutson DW. Multiple sclerosis: free light chains in cerebrospinal fluid. *Neurology* 1985; 35:1443-9.

[7] Link H, Laurenzi M. Immunoglobulin class and light chain type of oligoclonal bands in CSF in multiple sclerosis determined by agarose gel electrophoresis and immunofixation. *Ann Neurol.* 1979;6:107–10.

[8] Bracco F, Gallo P, Menna R, Battistin L, Tavolato B. Free light chains in the CSF in multiple sclerosis. *J Neurol.*1987;234:303-7.

[9] Sindic CJM., Laterre EC. Oligoclonal free kappa and lambda bands in the cerebrospinal fluid of patients with multiple sclerosis and other neurological diseases: an immunoaffinity-mediated capillary blot study. *J Neuroimmunol.*1991;33:63-72.

[10] Rudick RA, Pallant A, Bidlack JM, Herndon RM. Free light chains in multiple sclerosis spinal fluid. *Annal Neurol.*1986;20:63-9.

[11] DeCarli C, Menegous MA, Rudick RA. Free light chains in multiple sclerosis and infectious diseases. *Neurology* 1987;37:1334-8.

[12] Fischer Ch, Arneth B, Kehler L, Lotz J, Lackner KJ. Kappa free light chains in cerebrospinal fluid as markers of intrathecal immunoglobulin synthesis. *Clin Chem.* 2004;50:1809-13.

[13] Desplat-Jego S, Feuillet L, Pelletier J, Bernard D, Cherif A, Boucraut J. Quantification of immunoglobulin free light chains in cerebrospinal fluid by nephelometry. *J Clin Immunol.* 2005; 25: 338-45.

[14] Presslauer S, Milosavljevic D, Brucke T, Bayer P, Hubl W. Elevated levels of kappa free light chains in CSF to support the diagnosis of multiple sclerosis. *J Neurol.* 2008;255:1508-14.

[15] Katzmann JA, Clark RJ, Abraham RS, Bryant S., Lymp JF, Bradwell AR, et al. Serum reference intervals and diagnostic ranges for free kappa and free lambda immunoglobulin light chains: relative sensitivity for detection of monoclonal light chains. *Clin Chem.* 2002;48:1437-44.

[16] Bradwell AR. *Serum free light chain assays.* 5th ed. Birmingham: The Binding Site Ltd; 2008.

[17] Kaplan B, Aizenbud BM, Golderman S, Yaskariev R., Sela B. Free light chain monomers in the diagnosis of multiple sclerosis. *J Neuroimmunol.* 2010;229: 263-71.

[18] Gray HM, Kohler PF. A case of tetramer Bence Jones proteinaema. *Clin Exp Immunol.* 1968;3:277-85.

[19] Berggard I, Peterson PP. Polymeric forms of free normal κ and λ chains of human immunoglobulins. *J Biol Chem.* 1969; 244:4299-307.

[20] Solling K. Polymeric forms of free light chains in serum from normal individuals and from patients with renal diseases. *Scand J Clin Lab Invest.* 1976;36:447-52.

[21] Solling K. Light chain polymerism in normal individuals, in patients with severe proteinuria and in normals with inhibited tubular protein reabsorption by lysine. *Scand J Clin Lab Invest.* 1980; 40:129-34.

[22] Abraham RS, Charlesworth MC, Owen BAL, Benson LM, Katzmann JA, Reeder CB, et al. Trimolecular complexes of light chain dimers in serum of a patient with multiple myeloma. *Clin Chem.* 2002;48:1805-11.

[23] Wilkinson B, Gilbert H. Protein disulfide isomerase. *Biochem Biophys Acta* 2004;1699:35-44.

[24] Xiao R, Lundstrom-Ljung J, Holmgren A, Gilbert HF. Catalysis of thio/disulfide exchange. *J Biol Chem.* 2005;280:21099-106.

[25] Connors LH, Jiang Y, Budnik M, Theberge R., Prokaeva T, Bodi KL, et al. Heterogeneity in primary structure, post-translational modifications, and germline gene usage of nine full-length amyloidogenic k1 immunoglobulin light chains. *Biochemistry* 2007;46:14259-71.

[26] Solling K, Solling J, Nielsen, JL. Polymeric Bence Jones proteins in serum of myeloma patients with renal insufficiency. *J Int Med.* 1984;216:495-502.

[27] Kaplan B, Ramirez-Alvarado M., Sikkink L, Golderman S, Dispenzieri A, Livneh, A, et al. Free light chains in plasma of patients with light chain amyloidosis and non-amyloid light chain deposition disease. High proportion and heterogeneity of disulfide-linked monoclonal free light chains as pathogenic features of amyloid disease. *Br J Haematol.* 2009;144:705-15.

[28] Serafini B, Rosicarelli B, Magliozzi R, Stigliano E, Aloisi F. Detection of ectopic B-cell follicles with germinal centers in the meninges of patients with secondary progressive multiple sclerosis. *Brain Pathol.* 2004;14:164-74.

[29] Meinl E, Krumbholz M, Hohlfeld R. B lineage cells in the inflammatory central nervous system environment: Migration, maintenance, local antibody production, and therapeutic modulation. *Ann Neurol.* 2006;59:880–92.

[30] Lamers K J B, de Jong JGN, Jongen PJH, Kock-Jansen M JH, Teunesen M A, Prudon-Rosmulder EMW Cerebrospinal fluid free kappa light chains versus IgG findings in neurological disorders: qualitative and quantitative measurements. *J Neuroimmunol.* 1995;62: 19-25.

[31] Gallo P, Tavolato B, Bergerbrant S, Siden A. Immunoglobulin light chain patterns in the cerebrospinal fluid. *J Neurol Sci.* 1989;94:241-53.

[32] Goffette S, Schluep M, Henry H, Duprez T, Sindic CJM. Detection of oligoclonal free kappa chains in the absence of oligoclonal IgG in the CSF of patients with suspected multiple sclerosis. *J Neurol Neurosurg Psychiatry* 2004;75:308-10.

[33] Thio M, Blokhuis BR, Nijkamp FP, Redegeld FA. Free immunoglobulin light chains: a novel target in the therapy of inflammatory diseases. *Trends Pharmacol. Sci.*, 2008;29,170-4.

[34] Franciotta D, Salvetti M, Lolli F, Serafini B, Aloisi F. B cells and multiple sclerosis. *Lancet Neurol.* 2008;7:766-7.

[35] Redegeld FA, Nijkamp FP. Immunoglobulin free light chains and mast cells: pivotal role in T-cell mediatiated reactions? *Trends Immunol.*, 2003;24:181-5.

[36] Rocken M, Hultner L. Heavy functions for light chains. *Nature Med.* 2002;.8: 668-70.

[37] Rozniecki JJ, Hauser SL, Stein M, Lincoln R, Theoharides TC. Elevated mast cell tryptase in cerebrospinal fluid of multiple sclerosis patients. *Ann Neurol.* 1995; 37: 63-6.

[38] Zappulla JP, Arock M, Mars LT, Liblau RS. Mast cells: new target for multiple sclerosis therapy? *J Neuroimmunol.* 2002;131:5-20.

[39] Iwashita H, Grunwald F, Bauer H. Double ring formation in single radial immunodiffusion for kappa chains in multiple sclerosis cerebrospinal fluid. *J Neurol.* 1974; 207:45-52.

[40] Bollengier F P, Delmotte P, Lowenthal A. Biochemical findings in multiple sclerosis III. Immunoglobulins of restricted heterogeneity and light chain distribution in cerebrospinal fluid of patients with multiple sclerosis *J Neurol.* 1976;212:151-8.

[41] Laurenzi M A, Mavra M, Kam-Hansen S, Link H. Oligoclonal IgG and free light chains in multiple sclerosis demonstrated by thin-layer polyacrylamide gel isoelectric focusing and immunofixation. *Ann Neurol.*1980; 8:241–7.

[42] Krakauer M, Nielsen HS, Jensen J, Sellebjerg F.. Intrathecal synthesis of immunoglobulin light chains in multiple sclerosis. *Acta Neurol Scand.* 1998; 98:161-5.

[43] 43. Arneth B, Birklein F. High sensitivity of free lambda and free kappa light chains for detection of intrathecal immunoglobulin synthesis in cerebrospinal fluid. *Acta Neurol Scand.* 2009;119:39-44.

[44] Rudick, R.A., Medendorp, S.V., Namey, M., Boyle, S., Fischer, J., 1995. Multiple sclerosis progression in a natural history study: predictive value of cerebrospinal fluid free kappa light chains. *Mult. Scler.,* 1, 150-155.

[45] Rinker JR, Trinkaus K, Cross, AH.. Elevated CSF free kappa light chains correlate with disability prognosis in multiple sclerosis. *Neurology* 2006; 67:1288-90.

[46] Tate J, Bazeley S, Sykes S, Mollee P. Quantitative serum free light chain assay - analytical issues. *Clin Biochem Rev.* 2009;30:131-40.

[47] Briand PY, Decaux O, Caillon H, Grosbois B, Le Treut A, Guenet L. Analytical performance of the serum free light chain assay. *Clin Chim Lab Med.* 2010;48:73-9.

[48] Riberi M, Bernard D, Depieds R. Evidence for the presence of λ chain dimers in cerebral fluid of patients suffering from subacute sclerosing panencephalitis. *Clin Exp Immunol.* 1975; 19: 45-53.

[49] Kaplan B, Ramirez-Alvarado M, Dispenzieri A, Zeldenrust SR., Leung N, Livneh A, et al. Isolation and biochemical characterization of plasma monoclonal free light chains in amyloidosis AL and multiple myeloma: intact and truncated forms of light chains and their charge properties. *Clin Chem Lab Med.* 2008; 46:335-41.

Index

A

Abraham, 140, 141
access, x, 87, 102, 113
accounting, 132, 138
acid, viii, 12, 31, 35, 37, 39, 40, 41, 42, 43, 45, 46, 47, 48, 49, 50, 51, 52, 54, 55, 56, 57, 65
acquisitions, 117
acute infection, 105
acylation, 40
ADC, 116, 119
adhesion, 5, 36, 37, 73, 90
adipose, 55
adipose tissue, 55
adulthood, 82, 98
adults, 33, 83, 84
adverse effects, 73
aetiology, viii, 9, 31, 32, 38, 104
Africa, 32
age, 32, 41, 42, 60, 66, 67, 70, 76, 82, 83, 86, 98, 104, 106, 118
agonist, 74
AIDS, 133
albumin, 20, 40, 135
algorithm, 119
allele, viii, 59, 61, 84, 86, 105
amino, 11, 13
amino acid, 11, 13
amyloidosis, 133, 134, 137, 141, 142
amyotrophic lateral sclerosis, 95
anisotropy, x, 114, 117, 121, 122, 125, 126, 128, 129
annual rate, 73
ANOVA, 120
antibiotic, 40
antibody, viii, 2, 3, 4, 5, 6, 7, 8, 9, 10, 12, 13, 14, 16, 17, 18, 22, 24, 28, 30, 36, 60, 66, 70, 76, 82, 84, 85, 86, 88, 91, 92, 94, 95, 103, 104, 109, 110, 111, 112, 133, 134, 141
anticholinergic, 74
antidepressant, 53, 75
antigen, 2, 4, 5, 6, 7, 9, 10, 11, 13, 16, 17, 19, 28, 36, 38, 42, 65, 72, 73, 74, 83, 86, 91, 93, 94, 95, 99, 100, 101, 103, 106, 107, 108, 110, 111
antigen-presenting cell, 5, 6, 65, 72
antiphospholipid syndrome, 69, 78
anxiety, 75
APC, 5
apoptosis, 15, 29, 36, 64, 65, 77, 96, 100, 107
Aristotle, 59
aspartate, 64, 68
assessment, 34, 37, 115, 128, 138
astrocytes, viii, 5, 19, 36, 38, 43, 56, 60, 64, 72
asymmetry, 128
ataxia, ix, 33, 60, 68, 75
atoms, 41
atrophy, 64, 66, 68, 71, 78, 86, 96, 125, 129
autoantibodies, vii, 1, 4, 7, 8, 16, 18, 20, 23, 24, 26, 27, 29, 30, 65, 92, 108
autoantigens, 8
autoimmune diseases, 9, 23, 56, 61, 64, 74, 101, 106, 107, 133
autoimmunity, 9, 19, 22, 23, 24, 26, 27, 53, 75, 76, 89, 96, 99, 100, 107
autopsy, 68, 88
axonal degeneration, 114, 125
axons, vii, 14, 31, 32, 35, 65

B

bacteria, 11, 40
bacterial infection, 98
bacteriophage, 40, 56

barriers, 117
BBB, 63, 64, 72, 82, 90, 91
Belgium, 1
bending, 68
beneficial effect, 7, 73
benefits, 73, 74
benign, 53, 67, 78
bias, 125
biochemistry, 37, 53
biological markers, 22, 23, 27
biomarkers, 25
biomonitoring, 55
biopsy, 9
blame, 98
blood, viii, 3, 14, 16, 17, 36, 40, 42, 43, 48, 50, 51, 52, 53, 54, 55, 60, 63, 72, 82, 84, 85, 90, 92, 100, 102, 110, 135
blood stream, 36, 48
blood-brain barrier, viii, 50, 60, 63, 72, 82
body fluid, 47
bonds, 40, 41, 44, 133
bone, 2, 17, 63, 73
bone marrow, 2, 17, 63, 73
bowel, ix, 33, 60, 68, 75
bradycardia, 74
brain functions, viii, 31, 32, 125
brain stem, 68
brainstem, 69, 70
breakdown, 8, 61, 63, 125
Brownian motion, 115, 116
Butcher, 35, 50

C

C. pneumoniae, 62, 63
calcium, 5
candidates, ix, 14, 28, 29, 97
capillary, 135, 140
capsule, 101, 122, 124
carbohydrates, 40
carbon, 39, 40, 41, 44
carbon atoms, 41
Caucasians, 60
causal relationship, 111
causality, 79
causation, 106
CD8+, 55, 63, 64, 65, 72, 82, 89, 93, 99, 100, 107
cDNA, 9, 11, 12, 13, 28, 89, 90
cell culture, 13, 26
cell death, 4, 15, 38, 45, 65, 77, 107
cell differentiation, 7, 18, 21
cell division, 15
cell line, 10, 13, 14, 15, 16, 19, 29, 30, 77, 82, 95
cell lines, 13, 14, 15, 16, 29, 30, 77, 82, 95
cell membranes, 39, 42, 44, 47, 48, 53
cell signaling, 42
cell surface, 5, 6, 14, 17, 26, 36
central nervous system, vii, viii, ix, xi, 1, 2, 18, 19, 31, 32, 59, 60, 72, 81, 82, 94, 95, 97, 99, 128, 131, 132, 140, 141
cerebrospinal fluid, ix, x, 3, 18, 20, 21, 22, 23, 24, 25, 26, 27, 28, 29, 34, 54, 60, 64, 78, 85, 94, 102, 105, 108, 109, 110, 131, 132, 133, 139, 140, 141, 142
cerebrum, 127
chemical, 15, 36, 41
chemicals, 36
chemokines, 5, 63, 64, 65, 94
Chemotherapeutics, 79
childhood, 37, 67, 71, 82, 83, 98, 101
children, 33, 60, 68, 83, 91, 95, 109, 110
China, 111
cholesterol, 39, 44, 45, 46, 48
choline, 39
chromatography, 11
chromosomal instability, 15
chromosome, 39, 61, 133
chronic lymphocytic leukemia, 112
circulation, 5, 8, 100
CIS, 3, 16, 67, 68, 74, 86, 87, 114, 125, 138
classes, 36
classification, viii, 60, 66
clinical application, 117
clinical examination, 68
clinical symptoms, 69, 85, 86
clinical trials, 73, 91
clone, 86
clonus, 74
cluster analysis, 51
cluster of differentiation, 5
clustering, 61
CNS, vii, viii, 1, 2, 3, 4, 5, 6, 7, 8, 9, 18, 19, 21, 22, 32, 33, 36, 39, 42, 43, 48, 59, 60, 61, 62, 63, 64, 65, 66, 69, 70, 71, 72, 73, 74, 82, 87, 88, 89, 90, 91, 94, 99, 100, 101, 110, 132, 133, 134, 135, 139
cognitive deficit, 126
cognitive deficits, 126
cognitive dysfunction, 75
cognitive impairment, ix, 33, 60, 66, 68, 75
cognitive tasks, 33
collagen, 12
collateral, 101
collateral damage, 101
commissure, 119
community, 50

complement, xi, 4, 6, 7, 26, 131, 139
complementary DNA, 9
complexity, xi, 12, 13, 126, 131
composition, 11, 13, 39, 40, 42, 44, 45, 46, 48, 49, 50, 52, 53, 54, 56, 57
compounds, 8, 15
conference, 76
connectivity, x, 114, 117, 126
consensus, 11, 20, 78, 139
constipation, 75
constituents, 42
construction, 12, 13, 135
consumption, 41, 50
control group, 135, 138
controlled trials, 35
controversial, 68
COOH, 55
cooling, 74
coordination, 33, 68
corpus callosum, x, 114, 121, 122, 125, 126, 129
correlation, ix, x, 23, 26, 79, 81, 108, 113, 114, 115, 120, 122, 125
correlation coefficient, 122
correlations, 23, 48, 53, 121, 122, 125, 129
cortex, 66, 68
corticosteroids, ix, 34, 60, 71, 73
corticotropin, 63
cost, 60
costimulatory signal, 6
counterbalance, 74
covering, 88, 104
CRP, 37
crystalline, 13, 45
cure, vii, ix, 31, 32, 34, 60, 71, 76
cyclooxygenase, 56
cyclophosphamide, 34, 73
cyclosporine, 73
cysteine, 55
cystine, 55
cytokines, viii, 5, 6, 7, 19, 36, 39, 46, 47, 60, 63, 65, 77, 100
cytomegalovirus, 12, 13, 82
cytotoxic agents, 73
cytotoxicity, 4, 6, 15, 55, 64

D

daily living, 75
data analysis, 137
database, 102
defects, 101
defence, viii, 31
deficiency, 44
deficit, 68, 98, 126
deformability, 45, 55
degenerate, 107
degradation, 88
Delta, 41
dementia, 68
demyelinating disease, viii, ix, 18, 21, 22, 54, 59, 67, 68, 69, 70, 97
demyelination, vii, viii, ix, 3, 7, 12, 13, 21, 31, 32, 49, 59, 60, 62, 64, 65, 66, 68, 72, 77, 90, 97, 103, 105, 108, 114, 115, 117, 132
dendritic cell, viii, 5, 6, 7, 36, 60, 64, 65, 88, 132
Denmark, 98
deoxyribonucleic acid, 8
deposition, 133, 137, 141
deposits, 7
depression, 33, 53, 75
derivatives, 54
destruction, 13, 132
detectable, 8
detection, 13, 90, 103, 105, 115, 139, 140, 142
developed countries, 33
developing countries, 32
diabetes, 49, 53, 56
diagnostic criteria, 6, 20, 34, 69, 78, 85, 127
diagnostic markers, xi, 131
diet, 40, 41, 55, 62, 75
dietary fat, 35, 40, 42
dietary intake, 35, 42, 51
differential diagnosis, 68
diffraction, 45, 50
diffusion, x, 68, 114, 115, 116, 117, 119, 120, 125, 128, 129
diffusion-weighted imaging, 116
diffusivities, x, 114, 118, 125
diffusivity, x, 114, 117, 121, 122, 125, 126, 129
dimerization, 133, 137, 139
diploid, 15
diplopia, 68
disability, ix, 34, 53, 60, 66, 67, 68, 70, 71, 73, 74, 78, 81, 82, 86, 97, 115, 118, 135, 142
disability progression, 68, 74, 115
disease activity, ix, 3, 34, 74, 81, 92, 96, 109, 111
disease progression, x, 18, 35, 37, 39, 43, 49, 51, 53, 72, 114
diseases, xi, 9, 13, 20, 34, 38, 48, 49, 61, 63, 68, 69, 70, 84, 85, 87, 89, 98, 99, 101, 103, 109, 114, 127, 131, 132, 135, 138, 139, 140
disorder, viii, 2, 32, 53, 54, 59, 60, 61
displacement, 116, 118
distribution, 2, 3, 4, 33, 127, 142
diversity, x, 9, 13, 14, 20, 71, 97

DNA, 8, 10, 11, 14, 15, 23, 26, 30, 54, 83, 85, 90, 94, 102, 104, 105, 110
DNA polymerase, 83
docosahexaenoic acid, 41
DOI, 52, 53
donors, 82, 133
double bonds, 41, 44
drugs, 30, 34, 74
DWI, 116, 117, 128
dysarthria, 75
dysphagia, 75

E

EBV infection, ix, 38, 81, 82, 83, 84, 85, 87, 88, 89, 90, 91, 98, 99, 100, 102, 103, 104, 105
economic status, 83, 98
edema, 74, 116
editors, 27
EDSS, 34, 35, 43, 48, 53, 67, 68, 73, 78, 118, 120, 121, 122, 125, 135
eicosapentaenoic acid, 41, 50
electron, 45, 133
electrophoresis, 11, 69, 132, 135, 136, 139, 140
ELISA, 14
elongation, 47
elucidation, vii, 1, 16, 134
emergency, 83
encephalomyelitis, 17, 21, 67, 70, 78
encoding, 11, 130
endothelial cells, 5, 19, 76, 90, 91, 92, 93, 96
endothelium, 90
enemas, 75
energy, 39
environment, 15, 18, 39, 44, 57, 62, 106, 141
environmental conditions, 38, 133
environmental effects, 53
environmental factors, viii, 38, 59, 61, 62, 82
enzyme, 15, 29, 42, 44, 46, 64
enzymes, 4, 42, 46, 133
EPA, 41
epidemiology, 98
epithelial cells, 82, 90
Epstein Barr, 93, 95, 96, 107
Epstein-Barr virus, vii, viii, ix, x, 5, 20, 21, 22, 24, 27, 28, 29, 30, 37, 59, 62, 63, 76, 81, 82, 83, 91, 92, 93, 94, 95, 96, 97, 98, 102, 106, 107, 108, 109, 110, 111, 112
equipment, 136
erythrocytes, 51, 52, 53
ESR, 45
essential fatty acids, 41, 44, 46, 52, 53, 56
ethnic groups, 32
etiology, 16, 32, 52, 61, 82, 96
eukaryotic, 40, 52
eukaryotic cell, 40
Europe, 32, 33
evidence, vii, ix, x, 1, 2, 6, 7, 40, 61, 62, 65, 76, 81, 82, 83, 87, 88, 89, 91, 92, 93, 97, 98, 102, 106, 111, 115, 128, 130
evoked potential, ix, 34, 60, 68
evolution, 49, 114
examinations, 119
excitotoxicity, 64
exclusion, 66, 102
exercise, 75
experimental autoimmune encephalomyelitis (EAE), 2, 7, 19, 21, 61, 64, 74, 77
exposure, 36, 37, 71, 73, 76, 98, 103, 104
extraction, 120

F

Fabry disease, 70
false negative, 90
false positive, 90
fat, 40, 51, 56, 57
fat intake, 56
fatty acids, vii, viii, 31, 35, 39, 40, 41, 42, 43, 44, 46, 47, 48, 49, 50, 51, 52, 53, 54, 55, 56
FDA, 73
fever, 36, 71
fiber, x, 75, 114, 117, 125, 128
fibers, 116, 117, 128
fixation, 4, 88
flexibility, 45
fluid, 18, 20, 25, 41, 44, 45, 68, 75, 87, 93, 107, 108, 140, 141, 142
fluorescence, 45
follicle, 21, 134
follicles, ix, 5, 7, 18, 21, 64, 65, 81, 88, 89, 91, 100, 139, 141
food, 56
formation, vii, 5, 21, 31, 32, 36, 39, 42, 90, 100, 133, 142
fragility, 53
fragments, 37, 105
France, 113
free radicals, 65
freedom, 102, 117
functional MRI, 126
fusion, 12, 27

G

gadolinium, 66, 68, 115, 119
gamma globulin, 20
gastrin, 63
gastrointestinal tract, 63
gel, 11, 45, 132, 139, 140, 142
gene regulation, 56
genes, viii, 6, 13, 16, 17, 38, 57, 59, 61, 62, 63, 84, 88, 100, 108
genetic background, 7
genetic defect, 100
genetic factors, 38, 51, 104
genetic marker, 85
genetic predisposition, 99
genome, 11, 12, 85
genotype, 11
Georgia, v, 59
glatiramer acetate, 34, 73
glaucoma, 76, 77
glia, 54, 65
glial cells, 43, 49
glioma, 70
glutamate, 38, 43, 49, 55, 74
glycerol, 39
glycoproteins, 10, 11
gray matter, viii, 24, 26, 60, 66
Greece, 59, 76
group characteristics, 118
grouping, 122
growth, 15, 19, 63
growth factor, 19, 63
guidelines, 20, 78, 127

H

H. pylori, 62
headache, 73
healing, 36, 48
health, viii, x, 31, 32, 40, 48, 57, 98, 102
health care, x, 98, 102
heat shock protein, 26
Helicobacter pylori, viii, 59, 62, 63, 76, 77
hemolytic anemia, 70
hepatic encephalopathy, 70
herpes, viii, 12, 37, 54, 59, 61, 63, 82
herpes simplex, 12, 82
herpes virus, viii, 37, 54, 59, 61, 63
herpesviruses, 83, 85, 94, 110
heterogeneity, 9, 13, 16, 71, 128, 141, 142
histamine, 63
histogram, 129
histology, 127
history, 71, 75, 78, 83, 92, 98, 105, 118, 127, 142
HIV, 70
HLA, 61, 84, 87, 93, 94, 99, 104, 105, 108, 109, 112
homeostasis, 90
homogeneity, 115
hospital death, 52
host, viii, 11, 59, 61, 62, 63, 83, 112
House, 53
HSCT, 74
human, viii, 9, 12, 13, 14, 15, 16, 17, 18, 19, 22, 29, 30, 37, 38, 39, 41, 42, 55, 59, 63, 76, 77, 84, 90, 92, 93, 95, 96, 101, 102, 107, 109, 110, 116, 130, 140
human brain, 9, 13, 38, 41, 55, 76, 90, 92, 116, 130
human genome, 38
human leukocyte antigen, 39, 84
humoral immunity, 15, 20, 21, 36
Hunter, 32, 53, 91, 109
hybridization, 88, 89
hydrogen, 133
hydrogen bonds, 133
hydrolysis, 48
hygiene, x, 97, 98, 101, 109
hypertension, 73
hypothesis, x, 50, 87, 96, 97, 98, 99, 100, 101, 109, 115, 118, 125
hypoxia, 38, 49
hypoxia-inducible factor, 38

I

ICAM, 5, 50, 90
identical twins, 94
identification, vii, 1, 8, 9, 11, 12, 13, 16, 38, 71
idiopathic, 69
IFN, 64, 73, 77, 87, 88, 89, 94, 107
IFN-β, 73
IL-17, 64, 65
IL-8, 63
image, 34, 119, 128, 129
image analysis, 128
images, 115, 116, 119, 120
immune function, 105
immune regulation, 19
immune response, vii, 1, 2, 5, 6, 7, 8, 9, 14, 15, 16, 17, 22, 24, 27, 35, 36, 37, 38, 46, 56, 63, 65, 84, 85, 86, 87, 91, 92, 93, 94, 96, 100, 101, 108, 111, 132, 134, 139
immune system, viii, ix, 19, 34, 36, 51, 60, 61, 62, 64, 72, 75, 85, 87, 97, 101, 105, 107, 109

immunity, 18, 36, 50, 87
immunization, 17
immunocompromised, 112
immunodeficiency, 103
immunoelectrophoresis, 132
immunofixation, 140, 142
immunoglobulin, vii, ix, x, 1, 3, 6, 7, 17, 19, 39, 60, 62, 71, 108, 131, 132, 133, 135, 140, 141, 142
immunoglobulins, 65, 140
immunohistochemistry, 14, 89
immunomodulatory, 61, 74, 79
immunoprecipitation, 14
immunoreactivity, 5
immunosuppression, 72, 74
immunosuppressive drugs, 34
impairments, 75, 85, 115
improvements, 132
in situ hybridization, 89
in vitro, 19, 22, 26, 40, 101
in vivo, 9, 11, 13, 14, 15, 26, 52, 91, 109, 128
incidence, 32, 60, 98, 101, 111
individuals, vii, ix, 1, 2, 3, 9, 38, 52, 67, 81, 82, 84, 86, 90, 91, 99, 112, 140
induction, 7, 36, 49, 62, 63, 65, 74, 107
infection, x, 11, 15, 20, 29, 36, 37, 38, 53, 63, 71, 73, 76, 77, 82, 83, 88, 89, 90, 91, 92, 94, 95, 96, 97, 98, 99, 100, 102, 103, 104, 105, 106, 108, 112
infectious mononucleosis, 55, 82, 83, 93, 94, 95, 98, 102, 106, 112
inflammation, viii, 4, 18, 19, 22, 23, 25, 34, 35, 36, 37, 47, 48, 49, 50, 51, 53, 56, 57, 59, 60, 62, 64, 66, 69, 71, 72, 73, 76, 77, 90, 105, 114, 115, 118, 127, 132, 133
inflammatory cells, 100
inflammatory disease, vii, 31, 32, 38, 42, 82, 85, 132, 135, 141
inflammatory mediators, 53, 63, 134
inflammatory responses, 101
informed consent, 118
inhibition, 49, 56, 76
inhibitor, 73
initiation, ix, 7, 60, 62, 118
innate immunity, 36
inoculation, 63
inositol, 39
insulin, 49
integration, 34
integrity, x, 5, 39, 44, 114, 117
intensity values, 138
intercellular adhesion molecule, 5, 37
interferon, 19, 34, 39, 50, 64, 65, 79
interferon (IFN), 65
interferon-γ, 64
intervention, 57
intramuscular injection, 73
isolation, 86
Israel, 49, 105, 131
issues, 79, 89, 133, 142

L

laboratory tests, 136
latency, ix, 69, 81, 82, 86, 88, 89, 103
lead, 16, 28, 75, 87, 90, 125
leakage, 90
left hemisphere, 122, 126
lesions, vii, viii, ix, x, 2, 4, 6, 7, 13, 17, 19, 20, 21, 22, 28, 31, 32, 34, 47, 48, 54, 55, 60, 61, 64, 65, 66, 68, 71, 76, 77, 78, 86, 88, 89, 90, 100, 101, 114, 115, 117, 125, 127, 128, 129
leukotrienes, 36
LFA, 5
liberation, 100
lifetime, 32
ligand, 4, 5, 20
light, vii, xi, 10, 14, 131, 132, 133, 134, 137, 139, 140, 141, 142
linoleic acid, viii, 31, 41, 46
lipid metabolism, 42
lipid peroxidation, 56
lipids, 9, 10, 25, 39, 42, 44, 45, 48, 49, 51, 52, 53, 57
lipoproteins, 40, 53
liver, 55, 73, 74
localization, 114
loci, 61, 76
locus, 61
loss of consciousness, 68
Louisiana, 57
low risk, 83
LTB4, 46, 56
lupus, 133
lymphocytes, 19, 29, 36, 48, 50, 55, 61, 64, 65, 69, 74, 82, 87, 90, 92, 101, 107
lymphoid, 2, 5, 7, 17, 21, 74, 82, 88, 100, 101, 134
lymphoid organs, 2, 17, 100
lymphoid tissue, 2, 74, 101
lymphoma, 19, 70, 88, 103, 111
lysine, 140
lysis, 4, 19

M

Macedonia, 59
machinery, 11
macrophages, viii, 4, 5, 6, 35, 36, 46, 48, 60, 63, 64, 65, 72, 132
magnetic field, 115
magnetic resonance, ix, x, 4, 34, 60, 64, 68, 78, 86, 128, 131, 132
magnetic resonance imaging, ix, x, 4, 60, 64, 68, 78, 128, 131, 132
magnetization, 64, 68
magnetization transfer imaging, 68
magnitude, 121
major histocompatibility complex, viii, 36, 39, 59
majority, 3, 88, 100, 133
mammalian cells, 39
mammals, 52
management, vii, 54, 71, 79, 92, 114, 132
mapping, 128
marrow, 74
Mars, 141
mast cells, 63, 65, 77, 134, 141
matrix, 4, 63, 64
matrix metalloproteinase, 4, 63, 64
matter, iv, 42, 43, 51, 64, 66, 68, 86, 89, 96, 115
maturation process, 2
MBP, 7, 8, 14, 83
measles, 37, 83, 85
measurement, x, 102, 114, 115, 117, 119, 121
measurements, 47, 116, 125, 126, 128, 141
median, 67, 70
mediation, 35
medical, x, 53, 92, 113
medicine, 53
mellitus, 49
membrane permeability, 44
membranes, 39, 42, 43, 44, 45, 46, 47, 48, 56
memory, 2, 3, 7, 17, 18, 19, 55, 88, 100, 126, 130, 134
meninges, 3, 4, 5, 6, 7, 18, 21, 64, 88, 89, 100, 134, 141
messages, 56
messenger RNA, 5
messengers, 36
meta-analysis, 79, 93, 102, 103, 104, 106, 130
Metabolic, viii, 31, 32, 39
metabolic disturbances, 35
metabolism, 41, 42, 47, 55, 57
metabolites, 37, 40, 41, 48
metabolized, 46, 47
methodology, 78, 85, 103
methylprednisolone, 71, 73, 79
MHC, viii, 36, 39, 59, 61, 65, 72, 86
mice, 21, 65, 89
microarray technology, 9
microorganism, 103
microorganisms, viii, ix, 59, 97, 98
microstructure, x, 114, 125
migration, vii, 1, 2, 5, 13, 18, 19, 50, 61, 73, 74, 77
mimicry, 28, 86, 96, 107
mitochondrial DNA, 64
MMP, 4
MMP-9, 4
modelling, 126
models, 7, 75, 90, 117, 125
modifications, 40, 133, 141
MOG, 7, 8, 14
molecular mimicry, 63, 76, 83, 88, 99
molecules, viii, 5, 6, 14, 36, 39, 40, 45, 52, 60, 63, 65, 90, 99, 115, 116, 133
monoclonal antibody, 14, 91
monomers, 133, 136, 137, 138, 139, 140
mononucleosis, ix, 38, 81, 82, 83, 91, 106
monounsaturated fatty acids, 39, 47
morbidity, 74
morphology, 20, 53, 100
mortality, 35, 74
mortality rate, 35
mortality risk, 74
mosaic, 17
Moses, 37, 54
motif, 4, 5, 11, 13
MRI, x, 4, 34, 51, 64, 68, 69, 71, 73, 78, 86, 92, 113, 114, 115, 116, 118, 119, 125, 127, 128, 129, 131, 132
mRNA, 5, 20, 93
multiple myeloma, 133, 134, 137, 141, 142
multiplication, 138
mumps, 82, 83
muscle relaxant, 74
mutation, 2, 15, 18
myasthenia gravis, 30
myelin basic protein, 7, 22, 23, 24, 83, 87, 93, 95, 96, 99, 106, 107
myelin oligodendrocyte glycoprotein, 7, 22, 23, 24

N

nasopharyngeal carcinoma, 86, 103, 111
natural killer cell, 36
necrosis, 37, 64
nerve, vii, 5, 31, 32
nerve growth factor, 5

nervous system, 20
neural network, 125
neural networks, 125
neurodegeneration, viii, ix, 59, 60, 68, 72, 77, 97, 115
neurodegenerative diseases, vii, viii, 31, 46, 55, 65
neuroimaging, 69
neuroinflammation, 18, 65, 76
neurological disability, viii, 59, 60
neurological disease, 3, 11, 12, 13, 22, 23, 24, 25, 32, 37, 78, 86, 87, 92, 132, 135, 138, 139, 140
neurologist, 82, 119
neuromyelitis optica, 69, 70, 76
neurons, 34, 36, 41, 55, 63, 65, 127
neuropathy, 76
neuroprotection, 57
neuropsychological tests, 126
neurotransmission, 42
neurotransmitter, 38
neurotrophic factors, 5, 7
neutral, 40
neutrophils, 4, 46
New Zealand, 33
nitric oxide, 37, 39
nitrite, 37
NMR, 115, 128
normal distribution, 117
North America, 32
Norway, 94, 96, 106, 107, 110
Nuclear Magnetic Resonance, 115
nucleoplasm, 30
nystagmus, 68

O

occipital lobe, 126
occlusion, 116
oleic acid, 40
oligodendrocytes, vii, 22, 26, 31, 32, 35, 36, 38, 62, 65, 66, 73, 101
oligodendroglia, 55
oligodendroglioma, 16
oligomerization, 133
omega-3, 35, 50
optic nerve, 68, 70
optic neuritis, 68, 71, 75, 110
organ, viii, 59, 61, 100
overlap, 9
oxidation, 133
oxidative stress, 63, 65
oxygen, 45, 48

P

p53, 15
pain, 33
parallel, 98
paraneoplastic syndrome, 70
parasitic infection, 101
parenchyma, 4, 64, 89
parenchymal cell, 36
parietal lobe, 126
pathogenesis, vii, ix, 1, 2, 5, 7, 9, 21, 26, 42, 47, 48, 52, 54, 56, 61, 62, 63, 64, 65, 68, 72, 74, 77, 81, 82, 83, 86, 88, 97, 98, 100, 101, 103, 104, 105, 129, 133, 134
pathogens, viii, 36, 53, 59, 62, 63, 91, 101
pathology, 7, 18, 24, 26, 49, 60, 65, 68, 75, 77, 115, 125, 127, 134, 139
pathophysiological, 22, 23, 27, 55, 77
pathophysiology, 63, 65, 69
patient care, x, 113, 114
PBMC, 14, 16, 43, 46, 47, 48
PCR, 14, 85, 88, 89, 90, 94, 109
peptide, 10, 11, 12, 13, 14, 28, 72, 83, 86, 87, 98, 99, 108, 109
peptides, 11, 12, 13, 28, 83, 87, 88, 96, 107
perinatal, 26
peripheral blood, 2, 3, 4, 8, 14, 15, 16, 17, 37, 43, 54, 74, 85, 104
peripheral blood mononuclear cell, 14, 37, 43, 54
permeability, 44, 45, 48, 91
pertussis, 94
PGE, 47, 48
phage, 9, 11, 12, 13, 14, 27, 28
phagocyte, 4
phagocytosis, 4, 36, 42
pharmacology, 53, 55
phase shifts, 116
phenotype, 3, 11, 61, 88
Philadelphia, 20, 93
phosphate, 10, 11, 24, 27, 29, 74
phosphatidylcholine, 10, 39
phosphatidylethanolamine, 39
phosphatidylserine, 39
phospholipids, 39, 40, 41, 42, 43, 44, 46, 47, 48, 52, 54
phosphorylation, 66, 77
physical properties, 57
physical therapy, 74
Physiological, 54
pilot study, 93
placebo, 73
plaque, 7, 40, 57

plasma cells, 2, 4, 7, 14, 17, 18, 29, 36, 55, 64, 91, 100, 132, 133
plasma levels, 43
plasma membrane, 39
plasmid, 14
plasticity, 130
platelet activating factor, 36
platelets, viii, 31, 42, 43, 46, 51, 52
PLP, 8
PMS, 33
Poland, 50
polar, 39
polar groups, 39
polarization, 45, 91
polyacrylamide, 11, 132, 136, 137, 142
polymerase, 87, 109, 111
polymerase chain reaction, 109
polymerization, 137
polymorphisms, 61, 84
polyunsaturated fat, 35, 39, 47, 49, 50, 52, 55, 56, 57
polyunsaturated fatty acids, 35, 39, 47, 49, 52, 55, 56
population, 3, 26, 38, 69, 74, 82, 83, 94, 95, 98, 104, 110
porosity, 118
positive feedback, 6
positive macrophages, 17
postural control, 75, 79
prednisone, 73
pregnancy, 61
preparation, iv
preservation, 72, 88, 89
prevention, 55, 72, 74
primary progressive multiple sclerosis, 33, 129
probability, 116
probability density function, 116
prognosis, vii, viii, 1, 38, 60, 66, 69, 71, 142
progressive multifocal leukoencephalopathy, 73, 79
pro-inflammatory, viii, 31, 37, 38, 46, 47, 64, 65, 82, 89, 90, 91
proliferation, 5, 7, 15, 20, 66, 88, 100, 107, 117
prostaglandins, 36, 47, 50, 56
protection, 101
protective mechanisms, 38
protein components, 11
proteins, 8, 9, 10, 11, 12, 13, 14, 16, 22, 24, 26, 27, 36, 38, 39, 40, 42, 52, 53, 55, 69, 85, 86, 89, 92, 99, 107, 108, 141
proteinuria, 140
proteolipid protein, 8, 22, 25
proteolytic enzyme, 39
proteomics, 9
protons, 116
psychiatric disorders, 53
psychiatry, 53
puberty, 98

Q

quality of life, viii, ix, 31, 32, 33, 60, 71, 74, 75
quantification, x, 114, 118, 125, 126, 132, 135

R

radiation, 124
RANTES, 90
reactants, 38, 49
reactions, 41, 115, 141
reactive oxygen, 65
reactivity, vii, ix, 1, 2, 7, 8, 9, 14, 16, 29, 81, 85, 93, 94, 95, 105, 107, 112
receptors, viii, 4, 5, 8, 19, 20, 36, 37, 38, 43, 52, 59, 61
recognition, 33, 36, 82, 95, 99, 107, 126
recommendations, iv
reconstruction, 117
recovery, 33, 79
recruiting, 89
red blood cells, viii, 31, 42, 50, 52, 56
regenerate, 34
regulatory agencies, 73
rehabilitation, ix, 60, 75, 92
rehabilitation program, ix, 60
relapses, viii, ix, 33, 34, 36, 37, 54, 60, 66, 67, 70, 71, 73, 74, 78, 85, 91, 111
relapsing-remitting multiple sclerosis, 17, 22, 25, 26, 50, 66, 67, 78, 79, 93, 130
relatives, 38
relevance, 8, 16
remission, viii, 33, 60, 61, 66, 67, 77
remyelination, 7, 22, 26, 34, 114, 117
repair, ix, 7, 13, 97
replication, ix, 37, 56, 63, 81, 89, 93, 103
requirements, 48, 102, 117
residues, 108
resistance, 65
resolution, 115, 117, 119, 126, 128, 139
response, viii, 6, 7, 8, 14, 16, 21, 22, 23, 26, 31, 35, 36, 46, 53, 60, 61, 65, 66, 68, 73, 76, 83, 85, 87, 88, 89, 91, 93, 96, 99, 100, 101, 103, 104, 107, 129
restructuring, 57
retrovirus, 12, 37, 49, 54, 55, 56, 108

retroviruses, 37, 38, 61, 101
rheumatoid arthritis, 23, 103, 111
right hemisphere, 122
risk, viii, ix, 32, 33, 35, 38, 57, 59, 61, 62, 73, 74, 81, 82, 83, 84, 86, 91, 93, 94, 96, 98, 99, 102, 103, 105, 106, 109, 110, 111, 112
risk factors, 84, 98, 106, 112
risks, 74
rituximab, 17, 22, 73, 91, 93
RNA, 85, 88, 89, 93, 94
ROI, x, 114, 118, 121, 125, 126
routines, 117
RR-MS, 87, 88
rubella, 82, 83

S

safety, 74
sarcoidosis, 69, 70
saturated fat, 35, 41, 47, 48, 53
saturated fatty acids, 35, 41, 47, 48, 53
scarcity, 32
schizophrenia, 53
scientific knowledge, x, 98, 102
sclerosis, vii, viii, ix, 2, 17, 20, 31, 32, 33, 37, 50, 52, 53, 54, 55, 56, 59, 60, 68, 75, 76, 77, 78, 81, 83, 92, 96, 97, 105, 106, 110, 111, 112, 127, 129, 132, 139, 140, 142
SCT, 74
seasonality, 106
secondary progressive multiple sclerosis, 18, 21, 25, 33, 78, 139, 141
secrete, 5
secretion, 4, 49, 133
sedimentation, 54
senescence, 29
sensation, ix, 33, 60, 68
sensitivity, x, xi, 11, 13, 45, 56, 69, 114, 117, 125, 131, 132, 135, 138, 139, 140, 142
serine, 39, 63
serology, 85
serum, ix, 6, 8, 9, 11, 12, 22, 23, 25, 28, 37, 38, 42, 43, 49, 51, 69, 81, 85, 94, 103, 104, 105, 132, 133, 134, 135, 137, 138, 140, 141, 142
shock, 8, 109
showing, 82, 138
siblings, 38, 86, 92, 110
side effects, 71, 73, 74
signal transduction, 40
signaling pathway, 53
signalling, 107
signals, 5, 6, 99, 108
signs, 7, 104
Singapore, 53
skeleton, 120
smoking, viii, 59, 62
social life, 60
society, 33
sodium, 132
software, 119
somatic mutations, 133
South Africa, 31, 32, 33, 51, 54
Spain, 97
spasticity, 33, 74, 75
species, 64, 65
specific surface, 10
spectroscopy, 45, 68, 77
spin, 45, 115, 116, 119, 128
spinal cord, ix, 60, 68, 132
SP-MS, 87, 88
stability, 23, 73
standard deviation, 118
state, viii, 60, 65, 103, 104, 126, 130, 133
states, 98, 103, 133
statistical processing, 114
statistics, 118, 129
steroids, 72, 74
sterols, 49
stress, viii, 14, 56, 59, 62, 63, 71, 77, 91
stretching, 74
stroke, 49, 116
structural changes, 117
structure, x, 44, 45, 48, 49, 53, 54, 86, 114, 125, 126, 133, 141
subacute, 142
subcutaneous injection, 73
subgroups, 49
substrate, 46, 126
success rate, 7
succession, 11
sulfate, 132
Sun, 22, 25, 29, 76, 129
supplementation, 35, 55, 57
suppression, 6, 73, 92, 109
survival, vii, 1, 2, 5, 19, 36, 61, 89, 100, 134
susceptibility, viii, 33, 37, 38, 39, 59, 60, 61, 62, 76, 109
symptoms, vii, ix, 31, 32, 33, 34, 35, 50, 60, 66, 67, 68, 70, 71, 72, 73, 74, 75, 79, 86, 94, 98, 103, 104, 105, 112
syndrome, 3, 17, 20, 30, 67, 69, 70, 79, 86, 114
synergistic effect, 73
synovial fluid, 133
synthesis, 21, 25, 40, 41, 46, 47, 54, 69, 92, 93, 100, 108, 109, 110, 133, 134, 135, 140, 142
systemic lupus erythematosus, 69, 70, 103, 112

T

T cell, vii, ix, 1, 2, 5, 6, 17, 19, 21, 22, 55, 60, 63, 64, 65, 72, 77, 81, 82, 83, 86, 87, 88, 89, 90, 91, 93, 94, 95, 96, 107, 108, 109, 112, 132
T lymphocytes, viii, 19, 35, 56, 59, 61, 92, 93
T regulatory cells, 61
target, 3, 4, 6, 8, 9, 11, 13, 14, 16, 21, 24, 26, 28, 35, 36, 45, 63, 72, 95, 100, 141
target organs, 63
T-cell receptor, 72
TCR, 72, 86, 92, 93, 107
techniques, x, xi, 9, 14, 61, 68, 103, 105, 114, 115, 126, 131, 132, 135, 137
technologies, vii, xi, 1, 2, 14, 16, 23, 131
technology, 8, 11
telomere, 29
temperature, 33, 45
temporal lobe, 126
testing, 23, 135
TGF, 46
therapeutic targets, vii, 1, 16, 18, 72
therapeutics, 71
therapy, vii, 1, 6, 7, 15, 16, 17, 19, 21, 35, 38, 54, 61, 71, 72, 73, 74, 75, 79, 91, 141
thrombocytopenic purpura, 70
thromboxanes, 36, 56
thymus, 30
thyroid, 73
tissue, viii, 4, 5, 6, 8, 9, 11, 12, 13, 14, 32, 36, 38, 40, 41, 42, 43, 45, 47, 48, 57, 60, 63, 65, 66, 70, 88, 89, 95, 102, 104, 105, 111, 115, 116, 117, 128, 132
TNF, 5, 6, 20, 37, 46, 63, 64, 65, 77
TNF-alpha, 77
TNF-α, 63, 64, 65
toxicity, 73, 74
toxin, 94
TPI, 11, 14
trace elements, 55
trade, 74
trafficking, 72, 134
transcription, 38, 89, 101
transcripts, 89
transducer, 38
transection, 64, 77, 126
transformation, 15, 30, 93, 100, 101
transforming growth factor, 46
translation, 11
transmission, vii, 31, 32
transplantation, 35, 51, 54, 56, 74, 79
transport, 55, 76
treatment, vii, x, 1, 7, 8, 9, 31, 32, 34, 35, 42, 49, 52, 53, 60, 66, 68, 69, 71, 73, 74, 75, 79, 91, 113
trial, 17, 74
triggers, viii, ix, 2, 60, 64, 71, 72, 81, 82, 132
triglycerides, 39, 40
tropism, 73
tumor, 5, 39, 56, 63, 64, 76, 107
tumor necrosis factor, 5, 39, 56, 63, 76, 107
tumorigenesis, 29
turnover, 50
twins, 111

U

United, 32, 33
United Kingdom (UK), 32, 33, 53
upper respiratory tract, 37
urine, 133
USA, 20, 50, 52, 73, 107, 112, 120
UV radiation, 98

V

variations, 61, 84
vascular cell adhesion molecule, 5
vascular diseases, 69
vascular endothelial growth factor (VEGF), 63
vasculitis, 69, 70
vasodilation, 36
VCAM, 5
vector, 14, 116
vertigo, 33
vessels, 90
viral gene, 100
viral infection, 100, 105, 106
virus infection, 106, 109
virus replication, 40, 50
viruses, ix, x, 12, 37, 81, 82, 83, 85, 86, 95, 97, 106
vision, 75
vitamin B1, 70
vitamin B12, 70
vitamin B12 deficiency, 70
vitamin D, viii, 59, 62, 74, 98, 106
VLA, 5

W

wages, 60
walking, 70
Washington, 14, 29

water, 115, 116, 118, 128, 129
water diffusion, 128
weakness, ix, 33, 60, 68, 75
web, 102
Western blot, 14, 132, 136, 137
white blood cells, 42, 43, 51
white matter, x, 36, 42, 43, 49, 50, 53, 57, 64, 66, 68, 88, 114, 116, 128, 129
workstation, 119
worldwide, viii, 59

Y

yield, 42, 127
young adults, viii, ix, 32, 59, 60, 97, 114